Practical Professional and Leadership Skills: A Guide for Health and Social Care Professionals

Practical Professional and Leadership Skills

A Guide for Health and Social Care Professionals

NORMAN SARTORIUS MD, PhD, FRCPsych

President
Association for the Improvement of Mental Health Programmes (AMH)
Geneva
Switzerland

SIR GRAHAM THORNICROFT BSC, MB BS, MA, MST, PhD, FRCPsych

Professor Emeritus of Community Mental Health
King's College London
London
United Kingdom

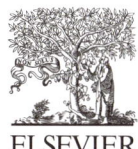

ELSEVIER

ISBN: 978-0-443-24877-1

Content Strategist: Robert Edwards
Content Project Manager: Fariha Nadeem
Design: Victoria Pearson Esser
Illustration Manager: Akshaya Mohan
Marketing Manager: Deborah Watkins

Printed in India

Last digit is the print number: 9 8 7 6 5 4 3 2 1

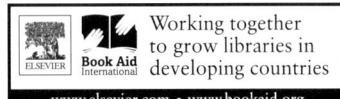

CONTENTS

SECTION C Skills Needed to Work Well Alone 165

Franziska Baessler, Dorota Frydecka, Ali Zafar Rizvi, and Olena Zhabenko, in association with Graham Thornicroft and Norman Sartorius

This **Practical Professional and Leadership Skills** book is grounded in the leadership course that Professor Norman Sartorius established and which has had a positive influence worldwide. Many course participants have later described that the connections they made with colleagues have developed into cherished friendships over the following years. No matter who you ask, most participants express their gratitude and describe how the course carried an immense value not only in their academic career but also their personal and social lives. These highly acclaimed courses-cum-workshops enhance the communication skills of young psychiatrists and facilitate their professional development by training them to use professional skills, by making them aware of their abilities and by supporting collaborative projects. In this Preface, we offer an appreciation of the lasting value and relevance derived from this teaching, instruction, guidance and wisdom.

Professor Sartorius, Professor Thornicroft and other teachers who offer the courses recognise the need for young professionals to develop competencies in areas such as scientific writing and reading, preparing and presenting academic work, learning how to work with others, navigating complex career challenges, writing research proposals, preparing CVs/resumes, speaking convincingly and listening, as well as learning how to assess priorities at work and in their development. These courses are now well-known for their hands-on approach and focus on essential, practical leadership skills, tailored specifically for professionals early in their careers.

Since the inaugural leadership course in Bangalore in 1992, many courses across the world have followed with participants coming from all over the world, creating a global community of course 'graduates', ready to assume dynamic leadership roles. Sixteen participants attend each course, and often there are over 100 applications for selection. Based on the popularity and success of these workshops among the global psychiatry community, a number of institutions and independent multinational groups have hosted courses – in some instances annually over the past 10 (India) and 20 (Japan and Germany) years.

Many participants of these courses have gone on to achieve notable careers and have shared their positive experiences about this leadership training. For example, alumni such as Anersha Pillay from South Africa and Chandrima Naskar from India have already written about how the course has shaped their leadership abilities, improved their communication skills, and empowered them to engage in mental health advocacy (Naskar and Varadharajan, 2024). These participants highlighted how the intensive, interactive nature of the course altered their professional perspectives and helped them network with other rising leaders in their professional field. Their reflections emphasise the importance of leadership skills that go beyond their clinical training, particularly in navigating complex health care or social systems and promoting health care reform in their respective countries.

The course on which this book is based has garnered a reputation for its unique approach, blending technical skill-building alongside leadership training. For over three decades, it has produced a cohort of early-career professionals who have gone on to make significant contributions to psychiatry and other fields, whether in academia, clinical practice, advocacy or policy.

Many course participants have found the course to be a transformative experience, recognising gaps in their leadership skills that the course uniquely addressed, with a particular focus on 'soft skills' such as communication across national and age groups, scientific writing, and presenting their work and themselves, that have been invaluable to their academic careers ever since. It is particularly the participatory, interactive nature of many skill-building sessions, such as pitching ideas or being interviewed for grant or fellowship applications, that have helped participants to build confidence and expertise and establish lasting friendships. Many former participants have gone on to become professors, involved with major projects and international collaborations, and the lessons learned from the leadership course continue to be relevant. In this Preface, the first three authors offer brief, personal appreciations of the value of this teaching.

Franziska Baessler

I participated in the leadership course in 2011 in Riga, Latvia, together with Olga Kazakova, who was co-organising the workshop. I still remember it vividly because for me it was an excellent experience where a lot of friendships and fruitful collaborations started. Olga and I have been friends and colleagues since then, organising different international congresses, conducting research together and volunteering in different organisations together. Also, we attended each other's weddings and we each have three children, so we share a lot in our personal lives.

I attended the course when I was a trainee in psychiatry, and I recall there was still much more to learn. I benefited immensely from learning about career-related professional skills, particularly on how to present a lecture, how to prepare for and conduct a meeting, how to write a report of a session, how to write a research paper, and how to read a research article. I also found the teaching of skills related to setting or assessing work and life priorities extremely useful in my career as a researcher and later as a project leader.

I remember acquiring valuable information about mental health care such as assessment of needs care and methods of evaluation of the outcomes of care. The course content was quite precise and was very interactively conveyed. We performed many role-playing sessions, such as chairing a meeting. One of the most valuable aspects of these sessions was the feedback we received, both from the teachers and from other course participants. At the end of the course, there was a vote, and I was voted most enthusiastic participant in the course.

At the course I attended, Professor Sartorius and Professor Goldberg from King's College London were co-teaching. There were numerous suggestions and recommendations from them on career development and networking, such as updating the master version of your CV at least once a year to develop a feeling about where you stand in terms of your career. Another valuable exercise for me was that you should take a group picture of your peers and label it with their names so that you can remember and recall everyone's names for a long time. Regarding posters, we were told always to carry copies of our posters with us in the A4 paper format with the authors' addresses, phone numbers and email addresses. Of course, due to digitalisation, a few things have changed over these years, so nowadays you need to learn the skills of how to make an e-poster and how to use social media.

For a long time now I have been fascinated by the effectiveness of these leadership courses. Together with Olga Kazakova, I initiated a qualitative study to explore the impact of these courses. Over the years, we have developed the study project, created an interview guide, piloted the interviews and conducted ethnographic interviews with many former participants of these Sartorius courses. During this time, several other colleagues have joined us (Olena Zhabenko, Dorota Frydecka, Marika Ganten) to work on this research, and we continue to meet.

What I consider to be a further important learning aspect of the leadership course is resilience. Our resilience was put to the test most recently during the COVID-19 pandemic. The pandemic-related restrictions significantly disrupted scientific gatherings and conferences throughout the world. However, we benefited from our leadership course network to organise a huge virtual gathering supported by the World Psychiatric Association in April 2021 (Baessler, Sartorius et al., 2021). This Train the Trainers workshop was cochaired by WPA President Afzal Javed and Professor Sartorius, who provided constructive feedback on each of the presentation sessions, where over 120 participants from 45 different countries convened (Baessler, Sartorius et al., 2021). I also created a video with delightful memories of the former course participants to present to Professor Sartorius as a token of gratitude and appreciation for his services in psychiatry.

Dorota Frydecka

There are several aspects of the leadership course that make it so impactful for young psychiatrists around the world. First and foremost, the course content covers the topics that are relevant for one's future career, but which are not yet incorporated into the regular medical curriculum. Secondly, the way that the course is organised allows the participants to establish very special and close life-long relationships that may last for years to come and are often the basis for future collaborations in research and other professional activities. And most importantly, the way that the course is led – with Professor Sartorius as the role model – creates this crucial impact, where it gives a sense of what it means to be a good leader. He conveys a special sense of confidence or self-esteem that translates into a feeling that ideas and plans that feel impossible to start at the beginning seem far more attainable in the future. In my experience, I had a feeling of being seen as valuable and accomplished although I was quite young and inexperienced at that time.

After the leadership course in which I took part in Berlin, I was invited to work as a guest researcher on the project *Artificial neural network modeling of reinforcement learning based on fMRI data* conducted at the Department of Psychiatry and Psychotherapy, Charité, Medical University of Berlin. The project was financed by the Bernstein Center for Computational Neuroscience, Humboldt University in Berlin. Later I was awarded a part in the *Mentoring* programme, financed by the Foundation for Polish Science (FPS), for scientific collaboration with Professor Andreas Heinz from the Department of Psychiatry and Psychotherapy, Charité Berlin, to continue our collaboration. Based on the knowledge acquired on the leadership course, I wrote a research project *Instructional control of reinforcement learning in schizophrenia: investigation using genetic data, behavioral data as well as computational models and artificial neural network models*, that was financed by the National Science Centre in Poland. In the project, I designed computer games that allowed investigation of the interplay between implicit and explicit learning among patients with schizophrenia and healthy controls, taking into account genetic, neuropsychological and clinical variables.

I later started a collaboration with the Technical University of Wrocław to analyse research data from my project using artificial neural networks and analytical computational models. This allowed for a deeper understanding of the interactions between the prefrontal cortex and basal ganglia, as well as how these processes translate to learning from rules and instructions on the one hand and environmental experiences on the other hand. Later, I received financial support from the FPS to continue my research on psychotic disorders *Instructional control of reinforcement learning in psychotic disorders (schizophrenia, schizoaffective disorder, bipolar disorder): investigation using genetic data, behavioral data as well as computational models and artificial neural network model*. I presented the results of my research in the science popularisation competition organised by the FPS and was awarded third place for my talk *Life (and mental health) as the art of decision making*.

From day one Professor Sartorius remembers all the names of the participants, respectfully refers to everyone as 'doctor', encourages deep discussions, allows all participants to play an active role in assessing one another in a constructive way, and gives a feeling that we are his equal partners and that what we say matters. This is very impactful as at the time of the course we are usually at the very bottom of the ladder, and at that time we were usually taught to be silent and follow the guidance, preferably without questioning, of more experienced colleagues at work.

This kind of approach has an especially important role in the context of learning how to give a presentation, which is a task that usually evokes a lot of anxieties and vulnerabilities related to public speaking. The detailed comments related to the strengths and weaknesses of our presentations were always fair, to the point, insightful, humorous and, most importantly, left us with a feeling that we actually can learn and do better in the future. We get the impression that we are not doomed by our natural skills, or lack of them, but that these skills are trainable and with the right feedback and effort clear progress can be made.

During the course, we had the sense that, as researchers and clinicians, our voice matters, and that it should be used wisely and professionally, because it is the main resource with which we can impact those around us. The course left us with the feeling that we want to pass on what we have learned, so that participants organise courses in their countries for their younger colleagues in turn. It is also very important that all participants are treated equally from the start. Despite coming from different countries, with different levels of research conducted at each university, participants have equal starting points. In the session about how to give a talk, the comments and feedback received were not about what was presented, but about how the talk was presented. During the course, Professor Sartorius was always focused, unbiased, kind, honest and respectful, and, surprisingly, seemed never to get tired of listening to our presentations. He treated us seriously, so that we could treat ourselves seriously. This approach was a big contrast to our usual educational systems, which focus on mistakes and failures.

Professor Sartorius has always encouraged an interdisciplinary approach, looking for inspiration from other disciplines and from collaborating with people representing different areas of research. He shared with us his life lessons about how not only to survive but also to thrive in an academic environment. Currently I am a professor in the Department of Psychiatry at the Medical University of Wrocław and also head the Department of Music Therapy at the Music Academy of Wrocław. I have also created a private interdisciplinary clinical centre where psychiatrists, psychologists, psychotherapists, neurologists, sexologists and dieticians collaborate to provide the best possible service for people with mental disorders. I have received numerous national and international awards for my research and served on many editorial boards of scientific journals, and I believe that the leadership course has played an important role in my success over the years.

Olena Zhabenko

The first three authors of this chapter are a group of former participants in the *Leadership and Professional Skills* course directed by Professor Norman Sartorius. My name is Olena Zhabenko, and I am originally from Ukraine. I am currently working as a senior psychiatrist with a subspecialisation in addiction psychiatry at the Center for Integrative Psychiatry, Psychiatric University Hospital Zurich, Switzerland. I participated in the Berlin Summer School 'Psychiatry as a Science – Genetic Neuroimaging' in 2009. It was my second unforgettable international experience as an early-career psychiatrist on that masterful, powerful, creative and unusual interactive leadership course. I had the opportunity not only to improve my presentation skills and deepen my knowledge in writing a CV and scientific papers, but also to interact with legends in psychiatry such as Professor Sartorius (Switzerland), Professor Heinz (Germany) and Professor Helmchen (Germany), as well as colleagues from all over Europe.

Over time, I met with colleagues at psychiatric workshops, seminars, conferences and other professional activities all over the world who had participated in the leadership course directed by Professor Sartorius (Mihai, 2006; Dumitru, 2017;

Baessler, Coskun et al., 2021; Baessler, 2013). After the course, we continued our collaboration in the IDEA-study (inpatient discharge: experiences and analysis) (Krupchanka, Khalifeh, Thornicroft et al., 2017), which improved our research competency over time, alongside other projects that originated in these courses (Krupchanka, Khalifeh, Abdulmalik et al., 2017). In 2014, Dr Costin Roventa and I received a grant from the Lundbeck International Neuroscience Foundation to help organise a leadership course directed by Professor Sartorius in Ukraine. However, because of the invasion of Ukraine by Russia in that year, the course was relocated to Moldova. Currently, our group is working further on a qualitative study investigating the experience of former participants who attended the *Leadership and Professional Skills* course directed by Professor Sartorius in Africa (South Africa, Kenya), Asia (Japan, Philippines, Singapore), Europe (Croatia, Latvia, Lithuania, Germany, Poland) and South America (Mexico). I am quite sure that the long-lasting positive effects of the course on professional and personal growth will continue to grow over time.

We close this Preface with further comments from other course participants to indicate the profound importance and impact of this course, and the topics covered in this inspirational book.

'This course is very important [because] I learn how to become a good leader. I still can recall his suggestions we need to be available, and he is a truly good role model.'

Dr Fransiska Kaligis (Indonesia), 2009
Singapore and 2012 Bali courses.

'It was a great life and professional experience, and we learnt so much.'

Dr Olena Zhabenko, 2009 Ukraine course.

'To participate in the course was a great pleasure and honour, and so we were able to have a fruitful career and start the Taiwan Organization for Young Psychiatrists.'

Dr Jane Chang, 2008 and 2015 Taiwan courses.

'The course influenced the lives of many people and since then fostered active collaboration.'

Prof. Elmar Rancans, course participant in 1995.

'Due to the leadership course we made fantastic friends. We feel privileged to call Prof. Sartorius our mentor.'

Dr Olga Kazakova and Dr Franziska Baessler, 2011 Riga course.

References

Baessler F., Coskun B., Pinto da Costa M., et al. (2021). Update from the Section Education in Psychiatry. Finding solutions: Training the trainers during a pandemic. WPA Review – Q2 eNewsletter. <https://mcusercontent.com/98a9ff0b264d6f7c78f9f1019/files/04606278-2feb-ec5a-8fa7-0e0d45831d0e/Section_education_workshop.kj.pdf> Accessed 25.07.21.

Baessler, F., Sartorius, N., Javed, A., et al., 2021. Training the trainers: Finding new educational opportunities in the virtual world. *Asia Pac. Psychiatry*, *13*(4), e12499. https://doi.org/10.1111/appy.12499

Baessler F., Zhabenko O., Tan L., et al. 2013. The Japanese Society of Psychiatry and Neurology (JSPN) Fellowship Award: Fostering International Collaboration Among Young Psychiatrists (in English, German, Japanese and Russian). News from Member Societies. World Psychiatric Association. <http://www.wpanet.org/detail.php?section_id=7&category_id=24&content_id=1432> Accessed 18.07.13.

Dumitru, M.M., Szczegielniak, A.R., Anastasova, Z., et al., 2017. The 16th Berlin summer school – psychiatry as a science and as a profession: Physical activity, exercise and mental disorders. *Psychiatr. Danub*, *29*(3), 387–388.

Krupchanka, D., Khalifeh, H., Abdulmalik, J., et al., 2017. Satisfaction with psychiatric in-patient care as rated by patients at discharge from hospitals in 11 countries. *Soc. Psychiatry Psychiatr. Epidemiol*, *52*, 989–1003.

Krupchanka, D., Khalifeh, H., Thornicroft, G., Sartorius, N., IDEA research group, 2017. Satisfaction with psychiatric in-patient care across 11 countries: Final report of the IDEA-study (inpatient discharge: experiences and analysis). *Eur. Psychiatry*, *41*(S1) S338-S338

Mihai, A., Ströhle, A., Maric, N., Heinz, A., Helmchen, H., Sartorius, N., 2006. Postgraduate training for young psychiatrists – Experience of the Berlin Summer School. *Eur. Psychiatry*, *21*(8), 509–515.

Naskar, C., Varadharajan, N., 2024. Beyond the couch: Empowering psychiatrists to be leaders – A brief report from a leadership and skills training course for psychiatrists in India. *J. Psychosoc. Rehabil. Ment. Health*, *11*, 135–138. https://doi.org/10.1007/s40737-023-00384-x

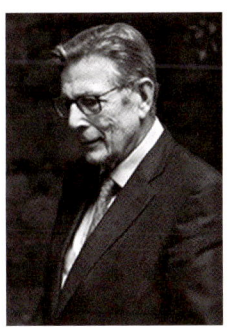

Professor Norman Sartorius
President
Association for the Improvement of Mental Health
Programmes (AMH) Geneva, Switzerland

Professor N. Sartorius, MD, MA, PhD, FRCPsych, previously Director of the Mental Health Program of the World Health Organization and President of the World Psychiatric Association and the European Psychiatric Association, now serves as President of the Association for the Improvement of Mental Health Programmes, a nongovernmental organisation located in Geneva. Professor Sartorius holds several professorial positions in Europe, the United States and elsewhere. He has published more than 600 papers in peer-reviewed journals, and authored, coauthored or coedited more than 120 books (with an h-index of 122).

Professor Sartorius' main areas of interest at present are the comorbidity of mental and physical disorders, the reduction of the stigma of mental disorders and the education of psychiatrists and other stakeholders in the field of mental health. In his previous positions he was the principal investigator of a number of international collaborative studies and projects dealing with schizophrenia and other major mental diseases, comorbidity of mental and physical illnesses, health service development and education of various categories of staff.

Professor Sartorius has received honorary doctorates from the Universities of Prague, Copenhagen, Bath, Umeå and Timisoara. He is an Honorary Fellow of the Royal College of Psychiatrists of the United Kingdom (UK), the Australia and New Zealand College of Psychiatrists and the World Psychiatric Association; a Distinguished Fellow of the American Psychiatric Association; an Honorary Fellow of the West African Postgraduate College; and an honorary member of numerous psychiatric societies. He is also an Honorary Member of the Medical Academies of Croatia, Mexico and Peru, a Corresponding Member of the Spanish Royal Medical Academy and Croatian Academy of Arts and Sciences, and a member of the International Academy of Arts and Science. He is also laureate of the Mahidol Prize for Medicine and recipient of a number of other prizes including Life Achievement Awards from the Royal College of Psychiatrists in the UK, the Croatian Psychiatric Association and the Asian Federation of Psychiatric Associations.

Professor Sartorius serves on the editorial boards of many journals and is currently one of the two main editors of *Current Opinion in Psychiatry*.

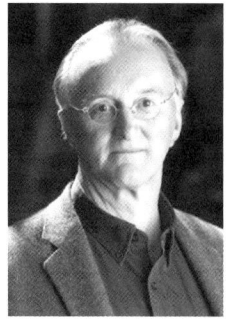

Professor Sir Graham Thornicroft
Honorary Consultant Psychiatrist
South London & Maudsley NHS Foundation Trust

Professor Emeritus of Community Mental Health
Center for Global Mental Health &
Centre for Implementation Science
Institute of Psychiatry, Psychology and Neuroscience
King's College London, UK

Graham Thornicroft, BSc, MB BS, MA, MSt, PhD, FRCPsych, is Professor Emeritus of Community Mental Health at King's College London. He is also an Honorary Consultant Psychiatrist at the South London & Maudsley NHS Foundation Trust, working in a local community mental health team. He is a National Institute of Health Research Senior Investigator Emeritus, a Fellow of King's College London, and an Honorary Fellow of the Royal College of Psychiatrists.

Graham studied for his undergraduate degree in social and political sciences at Cambridge, studied medicine at Guy's Hospital, London, and then trained in psychiatry at the Maudsley Hospital in London and Johns Hopkins Hospital in Baltimore. He gained an MSc in Epidemiology at the London School of Hygiene and Tropical Medicine, and a PhD at the University of London. In 2024 he completed an MSt in creative writing at the University of Cambridge.

Graham has made significant contributions to the development of mental health policy in England, including chairing the External Reference Group for the National Service Framework for Mental Health, the national mental health plan for England for 1999–2009.

He is also active in global mental health. He chaired the World Health Organization (WHO) Guideline Development Group for the Mental Health Gap Action Programme (mhGAP) Intervention Guide (1st, 2nd and 3rd editions), a practical support for primary care staff to treat people with mental, neurological and substance use disorders in low- and middle-income countries. This has been used in over 100 countries worldwide. He chaired the External Reference Group for the WHO guidelines on the Management of Physical Health Conditions in Adults with Severe Mental Disorders. He has recently also chaired the Guideline Development Group for the WHO guidelines on Mental Health at Work. He co-chaired the 2022 Lancet Commission on Ending Stigma and Discrimination in Mental Health. In 2024 he co-led the writing of the WHO Mosaic Toolkit to End Stigma and Discrimination in Mental Health.

His areas of research expertise include reduction of stigma and discrimination, evaluation of community mental health services, and global mental health. Graham has over 700 peer-reviewed papers listed in PubMed, and has authored or edited over 32 books, of which seven are award winning. Since 2020 he has been named each year by Clarivate as among the most highly cited researchers in the world. He is Chair of the Board of United for Global Mental Health. Graham has appeared in the media including BBC 1, the BBC World Service and BBC Today radio programme, and in The Economist. Graham received a Knighthood in the Queen's Birthday Honours Awards in 2017 for service to mental health.

CHAPTER 1

Introduction

Welcome

We would like to warmly welcome you to this book about leadership in health, care and research practice. The **aim** of this book is to provide you with very practical information that will enhance your ability to be a leader in your field. This book is mainly **orientated** to the skills required to work well in university, clinical and social care settings, but many of the topics included here are also relevant in many other areas of professional life and human endeavour.

Life for young professionals has many challenges and rates of burnout are unfortunately high. The experience we bring to this book is intended to help you to be clearer about what you want to achieve in your working life, and to be able to learn, practice and improve the skills needed for you to achieve your goals.

Our Perspectives

We have worked over several decades in health services, research and university settings, not-for-profit organisations, and global agencies such as the World Health Organization. From many projects and meetings that we have taken part in over the years we have seen examples of both outstandingly fine and miserably bad leadership. We will use some of the examples to help you to learn.

One of us (NS) has convened and led **over 100 courses** in recent years on leadership for junior doctors. Each course brings together about 16 early-career colleagues with a small faculty of teachers. Over three intensive days, students take part in a series of mostly interactive sessions to learn and practice key leadership skills. Feedback from many students has meant that this course has been progressively refined and improved over time. This book is based upon our experience offering this course to students, and from what we have learned from students in turn. Some of these students have been kind enough to offer their comments on the course (see Preface).

The Structure of Chapters

Each chapter breaks down the specific leadership skill into component parts. We begin chapters by showing related chapters as many of the skills we discuss are interrelated. In many chapters we provide short examples of good and bad practice. Chapters end with a summary of the key points we hope that you will note.

Some chapters include a short section of references, sources and resources if you would like to go into that topic in more detail. Several of the chapters also include details of practical exercises which you can perform, for example in a teaching group, to make the key issues in that chapter come alive through experiential learning.

We hope that you will use this book as a frequently consulted resource. Perhaps you have to prepare a talk for a conference, so you can dip into Chapter 2. Or maybe at short notice you are asked to chair a meeting, and in this case Chapter 11 is likely to be helpful to you. Although you may find that much of what you discover in these chapters is relevant to you, you may disagree with some of our comments. So much the better, as you develop your personal and individual style of leadership.

What Does Leadership Mean?

When we write about leadership what do we mean?

Leadership describes the set of skills required by a person who can successfully motivate (or even inspire) and organise a group of colleagues to be an effective team to achieve specific goals. Strong leaders can identify these goals and communicate them clearly to colleagues; break down the whole task into component parts; structure the team to work in a co-ordinated way to complete these components; manage and overcome setbacks; and integrate these components into the completed whole tasks. In many settings the work is undertaken by teams, and so strong leadership is a critical attribute for team success.

Soft Skills

In addition to the more specific 'hard' skills described in the chapters of this book, we also suggest you pay attention to what are described as '**soft skills**', which cut across all the specific domains. These leadership skills include strategic thinking, time and project management, clear communication, coaching and mentoring colleagues, timely decision making, and flexibility in when and how task components are managed. A further important soft skill of strong leaders is the **ability to delegate** tasks to colleagues: to share tasks fairly within a team, and to stretch team members with greater expectations than they have previously had while providing them with the support they need to succeed.

Repeated Practice and Direct Feedback

If there is a **core and recurrent theme** in this book, it is our view that the best way to learn these leadership skills is through **repeated practice**, specifically supported by **direct feedback** which you seek, consider and learn from. For example, when giving a talk at a meeting, ask a friend or a colleague to attend and to give you frank feedback afterwards on what you did well and what you can improve. We find that a lifelong commitment to learning, especially from the feedback of others, is a sound basis for becoming a highly competent, and perhaps one day inspirational, leader.

Skills Needed to Work Well With Larger Groups of People

In this first main section of the book, we present a series of short chapters about a range of skills you will need to work with larger groups of people. Even if your training or work is mostly concerned with caring for, treating, studying with, or collaborating with individuals or small groups, there may also be occasions when you need to work effectively with larger groups of people. By large groups we are thinking in terms of groups with more than 15–20 members. An example is when you need to prepare and present a talk or a poster to a large meeting or a conference. It can be if you wish to be elected to a responsible position in your work or profession. It can happen if you are giving a press or media interview. The chapters in this section offer you information that distils our experience in these settings and provides advice on how to work well with larger groups of people.

CHAPTER 2

How to Make a Presentation or Give a Talk

Introduction

Making a presentation to others is a vital skill that you need to acquire then keep improving, to assist you in your career. Think of talks you have attended that have been fascinating or even inspirational, and how you feel about the people who gave these talks (and the opposite!). This chapter offers you practical information on how to make strong presentations to other people. Many of the suggestions concerning a talk to a group are also valid for presentation to a single person, your boss, a friend or someone who reports to you. This chapter also cross-links with the other chapters shown below.

RELATED CHAPTERS

Chapter 3. How to ask and answer a question at a meeting
Chapter 13. How to chair a conference session

Before the Talk

Identify **what you want to say**. This is perhaps the most difficult step. You need to be very clear in your own mind about what it is you want to communicate to others. Write down a few sentences or perhaps a paragraph that says what your central message is. Read this aloud to yourself. Then simplify your message and simplify it again. Try to express the central message in one sentence. Tell a colleague what you will talk about in a sentence or two and see how they react.

Decide whether any **visual aids** will help other people to understand clearly what you want to say. Remember that your audience will include people who have different ways of paying attention and learning – some will learn through words, some through pictures and images, and some through the sound of your voice. Aim to offer your messages in all these modalities.

Find out exactly **how much time** you will have to give your talk. If the meeting or conference information does not make this clear, contact the person chairing the session or organising the conference and ask. Do not arrive at the meeting not knowing the time limit for your talk.

When you have prepared your presentation, for example, with PowerPoint slides, practice giving your talk to yourself, or to a friend or family member, or with a video recording, and time your talk mercilessly. **Do not exceed your time limit: try to speak for 10% less than the time allotted**. The person chairing your session and the audience will love you if you finish early and hate you if you are still talking when you time limit is reached.

Consider whether you need a plan or **table of contents** for the talk as the first slide of your talk, after the title slide. Generally, for a talk of 20 minutes or less this is not necessary, whereas it can be helpful for longer talks. If you show a table of contents, make certain that you do not have more than five chapters – longer tables of content need an introduction and this can take too much time.

Remember that the audience will be particularly receptive to your message immediately after you have shown the title slide, in the first minute or two of your talk, and then again in the penultimate part of your talk. For example, in a 10-minute talk the **maximum audience attention** is in the second and ninth minute (see Fig. 2.1).

Visual aids should not require much explanation, and should shorten, not prolong, the talk. Each visual aid should be clear to the viewer without your explanation. Visual aids are not obligatory.

Remember that there is an important difference between the *conclusion* and *the summary*: the conclusion describes the main finding and it will have to be expressed in a sentence or two; the summary must remind the audience of the key parts of the talk. Keep in mind the following basic rules:

- Be sincere: try to avoid giving talks on topics that you dislike or that bore you: your talks about them will bore the audience too.
- Say why the audience should listen to you: in what way does the topic about which you are talking concern them (or should concern them)? Will the participants learn something that they can use in their work? Will you present something that is important to them and that they cannot find easily elsewhere?
- Remember Aristotle's rule that a talk should have three key characteristics: ethos, pathos and logos. These are the roots of persuasion. Ethos refers to the credibility or authority of the speaker and to the observance of ethical issues, pathos refers to the emotion with which you are presenting the issues (Do you

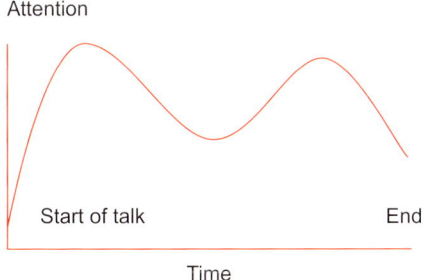

Fig. 2.1 Times of particular attention: early when you announce the theme and later when you present the conclusion.

believe in the importance of the subject? Does it really matter to you?), and logos refers to the logic, reasoning and your knowledge of the matter.

- Always finish on time or earlier.
- Be respectful of the audience: remember also that many of those listening know a lot about the topic you are addressing and many other matters.
- Dress appropriately (but comfortably).
- Do not be patronising, even if you do know a great deal more about a topic than those in the audience.

What to Check Before the Talk

Preparations and Checks Before Your Talk

- The location of the talk (building and room).
- The start time and end time of your talk and the session you are a part of.
- Who is managing the audio-visual equipment – say hello and make friends with them before the session.
- Who is chairing the session – meet and greet them before the session, if possible. Read up on their biography in Wikipedia or talk to people who know them. Sometimes it is useful to give the chairperson a note with your name and the topic of your talk on it.
- Check the meeting room before the session and familiarise yourself with the room layout, any obstructions for the audience in seeing you and the screen, the podium, the microphone, the PowerPoint remote control and any glass of water you may need.
- Remember Murphy's law that anything that can go wrong will go wrong and prepare for all eventualities – be a worried optimist.
- Remember that the quality of your presentation largely depends on the amount of time you spend preparing it (an old adage: 'if you fail to prepare, prepare to fail').

Present the material in your talk with emotion. Show that you believe in what you are presenting and that you think that it is useful and worth listening to. Within reason, the more emotion that accompanies your presentation, the more likely it is that people with remember what you have said (see Fig. 2.2).

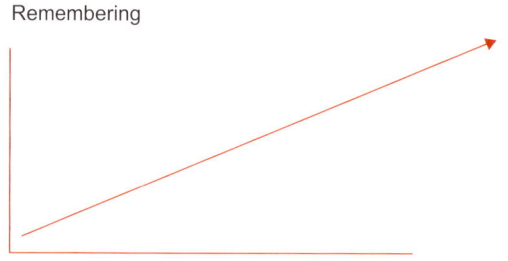

Fig. 2.2   The rational and the emotional.

Giving Your Talk

You should have been **introduced** by the chair of the session before you start. If you were not introduced to the audience, start with a very brief introduction to say who you are, where you work and what you do. Do not introduce yourself nor say your name if the chairperson has already done so: it will offend the chairperson, who will conclude that you did not listen to them or that you do not consider what they had said as being of acceptable quality.

When you begin your talk do not start with a joke. This can easily be misunderstood or backfire. If you feel that you must include a joke, do it later in the talk and make it a self-deprecating joke, that is, a joke against yourself. Start your talk with a short section to tell the audience what your talk is about and why you are making this presentation, for example, tell the audience that you will talk about an innovation in treatment which they might wish to use. If you have a relevant personal experience, use it in the introduction of your talk. State the importance of your topic in general and for yourself.

An example of **how not to start you talk**: *'I apologise for my poor English. I am keen to give this talk because I have been working on it for the last 2 years. We didn't get the grant for this work, but my friend had a word with the grant officer so the money came through late. I only have 10 minutes for this presentation so I will need to speak very fast. And what I really want to say is different from the published title of the talk, and this will be much more interesting for you. And now I need someone to help me to load my slides, if I can find my USB stick, which was in my pocket...'*

Key Points to Consider During Your Talk

- Do not apologise for any lack of fluency in the language you are using, your occasional cough, the bad audio quality or the quality of your slides – if you really see that any of these conditions are likely to make your talk incomprehensible or otherwise useful, do not give the talk.
- Do not say how difficult it was for you to prepare this talk.
- Always acknowledge others who have contributed to the talk, preferably at the beginning, and possibly with a photo of the group that worked on the project that you are presenting.
- Prepare and learn your opening and closing sentences by heart, so that you can say them without looking at your slides and while looking directly at the audience, seeking to establish eye contact with as many of them as possible.
- Try to maintain eye contact with your audience throughout the talk.

The Content of the Talk and Use of Slides

- Condense the key message of your talk into one or two sentences
- Give this key message at the beginning or the end of the talk
- Give each slide a clear and, whenever possible, short title and write it in large font

- Use a different title for each slide: try to avoid having several slides with the same title with a number following it (e.g., Other factors (1); Other factors (2); Other factors (3))
- Use few lines or bullet points on each slide (few or fewer), and preferably only one line of text for each bullet point
- For slide titles use at least 36-point font
- For main text in slides use at least 20-point font
- Give only the key references for a statement if that is necessary, by citing the author and the year of publication only, showing them in the right lower corner of the slide

Example of a Well-Prepared Slide

This slide has the following *positive characteristics*:
- Strong contrast between text and background colours
- Large font for the title text (36 point)
- Large font for the main text (30 point)
- Each bullet point has one or two lines only
- Only three bullet points
- Restrained use of bold font to highlight key elements
- Full text grammar is not used
- There is no punctuation
- The meaning of the slide can be understood from the title and the main text only
- The slide allows the speaker to elaborate by adding verbal detail

Example of a Poorly-Prepared Slide

This slide has the following *negative characteristics*:
- Small and essentially illegible font
- Poor contrast between text and background colours
- Too much information is included
- A title that is not clear – what does work package mean and work packages of what?
- Inconsistent use of colour – what do the different box background colours mean?
- Text that overlaps with other text and makes both text elements confusing

Tools to Use in Your Talk

You have a range of tools to help you to get your message across:
- **Eyes:** Scan you audience all the time during your talk and try to keep almost continuous eye contact with them. Look at your slides as little as possible. Practice so that you know the content of the slides before your talk.
- **Hands:** Move your hands moderately actively and in a symmetrical way. Do not let your hands move above your shoulders or below your waist. Do not put your hands in your pockets. Remember that such nonverbal gestures can connect more powerfully with your audience than what you try to say with words, and it will confuse the audience if the verbal and nonverbal messages you give are conflicting.

- **Legs and body:** Remember that the audience will watch how you behave during the talk. Do not move too much, and turn towards the audience and avoid defensive positions (such as crossed arms). Do not turn away from the audience – they should never see your back. Do not 'dance' – stay on one spot but shift your weight onto alternate legs.
- **Voice:** Speak slowly enough that all your audience can follow what you say and to allow any translator or interpreter to keep up with you. As you may be nervous about giving your talk, exaggerate a little how much you slow down your speech during your talk to compensate. Be sure to speak loud enough so that (with or without microphone and loudspeakers) everyone in the room can hear you clearly. Aim to be heard particularly well by those sitting at mid-distance; do not shout so that those far away hear you best.
- **Dress:** Show respect for your audience by dressing a little more formally and in the custom of the setting of the talk. Do some homework about what dress is usual, for example, go to a meeting at the conference the previous day to see what dress code is used.
- **Pointer:** A laser pointer can be helpful to draw the attention of the audience to a particular part of slide. When you use it, make it still on the screen and do not wave it in a vague circular pattern. If you are nervous and the pointer spot is shaking on the screen, use your other hand to steady the hand holding the pointer.
- **Microphone:** Hold the microphone near your mouth so the audience can hear you clearly, and keep it in the same position. Some microphones are directional and will only work well if you stand directly in front of them. Test this when you go to the meeting room before your session.
- **Lights:** The audience wants to see you, especially your face. If you can, arrange lighting in the room so that your face is well illuminated. At the same time, avoid direct lighting falling on the screen, which will make your slides less clear. You may need to close curtains or blinds at the front of the room to increase brightness and contrast for your slides. This underlines the importance of knowing your conference room.
- **Clock:** Have a clear sight of the time, how long you have for your talk, and how long you have left. There may be a conference timer, or use your watch or phone to show you the time.
- **Podium:** Go to the room before your session to check how to get onto the stage. Where are the stairs? How can you rise to the stage elegantly and without stumbling?
- **Lines of sight:** If you have a choice, stand in the middle of the podium, where all the audience can see you clearly. Are there any pillars or other obstructions you need to consider?
- **Handouts:** If you have handouts, announce this at the end of the talk and give them out at the end not at the beginning. This will ensure that the audience will listen to you, rather than look at handouts or pay little attention to you as they have a handout of what you are saying.
- **Blackboard and flipboards:** Using these sparingly during talks can be very effective if you make very simple and easily seen drawings and if you prepare the board and pens so that no time is lost.
- **Recording:** If a session is being recorded, tell the audience this, to provide information about any privacy concerns.

Mistakes to Avoid

Things Not to Do During Your Talk

- Do not apologise for your accent or use of a particular language, your cough, or your hoarse voice. If it is likely that you will not be understood because of any of these or for any other reason, do not give the talk.
- Do not be disrespectful of anyone.
- Do not claim a right to have more than your allocated time.
- Do not repeat yourself.
- If there is a sudden noise or other disturbance, do not stop your talk unless told to do so by the chair. If there is a power failure or the projector does not work properly, continue your talk without your slides – so always have a hard copy of your slides with you when you go to the podium to speak.
- Do not keep your phone switched on while you give your talk.
- Make an effort to speak to the audience before you and not to the audience you wished you might have had.

Using Slides

Key Points to Consider When Using PowerPoint Slides

In our opinion, slides such as PowerPoint slides work best:
- In landscape format only.
- Using three colours or fewer.
- Using plain font, without serif.
- If they are understandable in 10 seconds or less without your explanation.
- If they are not crammed. If you have more than four or five lines of text on one slide, move the additional information onto the next slide. Aim also to have one slide per minute of your presentation.

Remember – particularly in a short talk – it is better to have one line of text on each of two slides than one slide with two lines of text.

Using Prompt Cards

If you have trouble remembering what you plan to say in your talk, may be forgetful because of anxiety or nervousness, or cannot show slides accompanying your talk, it can help to prepare **prompt cards** or **notes on your phone or tablet**, to help you with your key points:
- Put just a few key words on each card
- Number the cards
- Write on your cards in very large letters, but avoid all text in capital letters because words are less legible when they are written with capitals only
- Put the cards in the correct sequence and tie them together with a ring so they will not lose their correct order if you drop them
- Use the cards when you practice the talk

■ Look at each card quickly for each point you make or slide, and mostly keep scanning the audience for eye contact all the time during your talk

The End of Your Talk

End your talk with a final slide with your contact details and thanks to the audience for their attention. Do not end your talk by inviting questions. The chairperson of the session will decide if there is time for questions or not and invite the audience to ask them.

After Your Talk

The work has not finished after you have ended your talk. Be sure to talk with the other speakers informally after the formal presentation has ended. Have your personal card to give out to them. Be sure to thank the chair of the session for their contribution to the success of the meeting. Be available for some time after the talk to receive informal queries or questions from members of the audience. Decide whether you want to write up your talk for a paper or other publication. One of the main aims of your talk is to make yourself known, and to initiate contacts and networks. You might therefore wish to write to those who were with you in the session, possibly send them some other publications on the same topic, or just say a friendly word about the congress and the time spent together. If anyone helped you with your slides or otherwise helped you to make the presentation, give them feedback, telling them what happened and how things went. Add details of the session to your curriculum vitae.

If friends or colleagues attended the session, ask them for honest and clear feedback about what went well in your talk and what could be improved in future. Take feedback about your talks seriously. Remember that you have learned something during the talk you gave and use the experience for the next talk you give.

Key Points

■ Decide clearly what you want to say
■ Stay on this topic and do not include other material
■ Understand your time limit and cut your talk content to fit this
■ Learn who your audience is and find out what they already know on your topic
■ Decide if you need visual aids and keep to guidelines on clear use of slides
■ Practice your talk with colleagues or with video feedback
■ Familiarise yourself with the venue before your session starts
■ Learn how to use the audio-visual aids
■ Seek feedback after your talk about what went well or not so well and learn

Practical Exercise

Before the start of the teaching course each member of the group is invited to prepare an 8-minute talk. No other information is given. Each member may or may not decide to use slides for the talk. During the course, several sessions are programmed for these talks. For each presentation, the member is invited to give their talk. A teacher times the talk and asks the presenter to stop after 8 minutes if necessary. Any time used for the presenter to set up the slide files, after they are invited to start, is taken away from their time allocation. After the presentation, the speaker remains at the front of the room. The group is invited to comment on what they found impressive or less impressive about the talk. The speaker is not allowed to respond or give defensive replies to the comments at this stage. The teachers then ask the presenter to show the slides again in sequence so that detailed comments can be made about specific strengths or weaknesses demonstrated on the slides. The members of the group are asked to make their comments in a neutral way, about the talk and the slides rather than about the person. Often teachers will use the 'sandwich technique', i.e., they will make a positive comment, then a negative/formative comment, and then another positive comment. Towards the end of the session the speaker is asked to offer brief reflections on the comments received. Detailed comments on each presentation can take 15–20 minutes. As the speaker sits down the group offer applause.

A variation on this type of practical exercise is for a teacher to sit down with the presenter in front of the group, and to edit, for example, four or five PowerPoint slides live in front of the class. While editing, the teacher indicates why they are making specific edits, for example, to the font type, font size, uses of figures or use of colours.

References

Conlon, J. D. (2023). *Essential communication & influencing skills: A practical guide to verbal & non-verbal communication. Independent publication.* ISBN-13: 979-8719336831.

Smith, R. (2000). How not to give a presentation. *BMJ, 321*(7276), 1570–1571.

CHAPTER 3

How to Ask and Answer a Question at a Meeting

Teaching or professional meetings commonly include a number of presentations, after which there is a 'Question and Answer' session. How can you prepare, to make these sessions useful for you? These skills are related to those shown below.

RELATED CHAPTERS

Chapter 2. How to make a presentation or give a talk
Chapter 6. How to behave in an interview with the media
Chapter 13. How to chair a conference session
Chapter 14. How to take part in a meeting

How to Ask a Question

If you are at a scientific or clinical meeting and hear a presentation, you may wish to ask the presenter a question. We suggest the following guidelines:

- Stand up to ask your question.
- If there is a microphone use it, and check that it is on.
- Start by thanking the chair for the opportunity to ask the question.
- Be polite and respectful at all times.
- The question should be a single (not multiple) question and be short. It should be directly related (and not indirectly related) to what was presented.
- Your question should be a question and not a statement in disguise.
- Your point must be objective and about the talk just given, and must not be a personal comment, especially not an offensive comment.
- Do not ask hypothetical questions.

How to Answer a Question

If you have given a presentation and now face questions from the group or audience, when you are asked a question try to understand why the question is being asked. It may be because the questioner wants to obtain more information, to promote themselves or to give their own message, or they may want to help you. In replying to a question, do not start by saying that the question is interesting or excellent. This can be understood to mean that the other questions you are asked are not excellent! After answering the question, do not ask the questioner to make further comments

('Does this answer your question?') because that might lead to a prolonged dialogue and take time away from other people who are waiting to ask you a question.

In responding to a query, do not avoid the question or give an answer to a different question. Admit it openly if you do not have the answer to a particular question. You can add that you would be pleased to meet the questioner after the session to discuss this issue further. You could also mention the name of a person who is likely to be able to answer that question.

Quite often you may not understand, or not fully understand, the question. This could be because the questioner is not stating the question clearly, or perhaps because the sound system or the acoustics in the room are unclear, or because the interpretation service has struggled to give a clear translation. You can either ask the speaker to repeat or paraphrase the question or, more usefully, turn to the chair of the session to ask for help to clearly understand the question. This also gives you a little more time to mentally compose your answer. This is better than guessing what the question may be about. If the questioner does not use a microphone when stating the question you can speak into your microphone to briefing summarise the question before you answer, and this can help the audience, either in the room or people taking part online, to hear both the question and your answer.

Before the session, practice with colleagues or friends and ask them to ask you very difficult questions, so that you have preprepared answers if they are asked at the actual event. Rehearse your answers to the most difficult expected questions. If you are asked a hypothetical question, it is usually acceptable to say that you are not able to answer hypothetical questions. Similarly, do not answer questions that are not related to the content of your talk.

Structure your answers to questions by using the **ABC technique (see** Table 3.1**)**. **Acknowledge:** the question and its importance. **Bridge:** make a link between the question and what you want to say. **Communicate:** add your main comment in replying to the question.

Key Points

- Before answering a question consider why the question is being asked
- Answer each question directly
- If you do not know the answer to a question, say so
- Do not say that any particular question is an excellent question
- If you cannot understand the question, ask the session chair to help you
- Practice answering difficult questions before the session
- Use the ABC technique to answer questions.

TABLE 3.1 ■ **ABC Technique for Answering Questions (Make Worksheet)**

Acknowledge	Bridge	Communicate
'This has been published…'	'But we also know that…'	Give your key message
'People believe this…'	'We are convinced…'	Give your key message

Practical Exercise

In the teaching group, ask for three volunteers for a practical exercise on answering questions. The teacher asks the first student to answer question 1. After the response, the group discusses what parts of the answer were strong or less strong. The teacher then gives an example of how to answer the question using the ABC technique, as shown below. Go on to questions 2 and 3 using the same method.

Question 1

'*Is it true that people with mental illness who come to your hospital are kept there unnecessarily, against their will?*'

Acknowledge: I have heard this being said and I have even seen it in the newspaper.

Bridge: I work at this hospital, and over the past 10 years I have never seen this happen.

Communicate: In fact, the law requires that a judge sees the patient who is brought in by the emergency services within 24 hours... (and you then continue by describing the law and good clinical practice).

Question 2

The husband of a woman being treated in hospital for depression asks the doctor how long she will need to stay in hospital.

Acknowledge: I understand that this is a difficult situation for the whole family while your wife is in hospital.

Bridge: It is very difficult to foresee how long the treatment will take for any particular individual patient, so I cannot tell you exactly.

Communicate: But what I can say is that on average people in our hospital with this condition stay in hospital for about 3 weeks before going home. I would like to stay in close touch with you, and to give you regular updates on your wife's condition, her progress and what to expect. And I will give you our contact phone number if you have any further questions.

Question 3

A patient asks the doctor if she should have children.

Acknowledgement: I can well understand the importance of this question for a woman of your age and how you need to take these issues very seriously.

Bridge: Of course, this is your decision, but as you have asked for my view I am pleased to offer this to you.

Communication: You only began to have mental health difficulties a few weeks ago, and this is an early stage in your treatment and recovery. I would suggest that you do not make a decision about having children at the moment but wait until you are feeling better and your recovery has been more fully established.

CHAPTER 4

How to be Elected

Many organisations, for example, the European Psychiatric Association, ask candidates who satisfy the criteria for a post to speak to the electorate for a few minutes. This is done because many of the candidates have similar qualifications, and it is difficult to select one among them. This chapter offers you advice on how to be elected. Several other chapters, as shown below, are also related to this topic.

RELATED CHAPTERS

Chapter 2. How to make a presentation or give a talk
Chapter 6. How to behave in an interview with the media
Chapter 10. How to present oneself to a group of people
Chapter 18. How to behave in an interview for a post
Chapter 21. How to make an elevator pitch
Chapter 33. How to write a letter of motivation (cover letter)
Chapter 37. How to apply for a post

A brief presentation is the main criterion for selecting one among the candidates. It is important to remember that the suggestions given here are *also usable* when you wish to express an *interest in being given a particular task* or mission while retaining your current position.

Please do not present your candidacy for a new position unless you are certain that:

- *you will not miss your previous position*, friends you have made, or traces of work that you have done and are proud of.
- you have *spoken to the previous incumbents* of this position or post about the difficulties and problems that they have faced.
- you have *talked to your family and friends* about your intention to present yourself as a candidate and obtained their views about that.

If you are invited to tell an audience why your *qualifications* make you the best candidate, you should remember that your qualifications often matter less than *the way in which they are presented*. Remember the **Penfield rule**: to drive the members of a group towards a particular decision, the person making a proposal needs to gain the support of the square root of the number of group members. For example, in a group of 24 people, one needs to gain the clear support of just 5 individuals to increase the probability of carrying the motion or proposal.

Key Points in Making a Good Case for Being Elected

- Try to be physically *fit for the presentation*. This might require that you postpone some other exhausting obligations so that you have a good night's sleep before the date of the election.
- Try to find out *where you will make your presentation* and whether it will have to be done with some *technical help*, for example, with a microphone. If you have a choice, *do not use a microphone* but come closer to the audience to speak to them.
- Start the presentation with a *cordial greeting* of the audience and a friendly expression. Address the rank and title of the electors.
- Start by a *description of the needs* to which the elected person will have to respond. Make the description as specific as possible. Do not say, for example, 'We all know that services for the elderly are insufficient'; rather say 'At present there are two wards for severely ill elderly people and only two nurses, who must look after all their needs, 24 hours a day'.
- The description of the needs should *focus on things that can be changed*.
- Describe any *personal experience* in relation to the needs, for example, that you have participated in a programme aiming to improve a similar situation. Be specific.
- Proceed from there to describe *what other skills or assets you have* (e.g., fluency in a language, previous experience and additional training) in relation to the tasks you have and *mention your qualifications* in passing.
- Describe *what you would* do if you were elected. Do not make promises about things that all know will be very difficult to fulfil.
- Try to *describe what the audience/electorate will gain* if you are elected. If possible, compose this part of your presentation on the basis of *discussions that you had with the electors before the election*.
- Spend some time describing what improvements you are hoping to achieve for *different subgroups of the electorate*.
- Try to *praise* the ideas of *those who might be reluctant to vote for you*.
- *Praise the work of predecessors*, or at least do not say bad things about them or their work: in your audience there will be individuals who have voted for your predecessor.
- Use the *rules of good presentation* given in Chapter 2– time yourself, try the talk on friends, and know it sufficiently not to have to look at any papers.
- Very importantly, when you *speak about problems, do so with a ray of hope* that they can be changed.
- Once the election is over, speak to people who promised that they will help and *thank them for their support*.
- Give a *smile and a handshake to your opponents* regardless of whether you have won the election or lost it.

WORKSHEET 4.1

Exercise

Three participants in the group are asked to volunteer. The task is to stand before the group and to make a short speech or pitch on why they should be elected for a relevant important position, such as the head of an association. In turn, each person makes a formal 2-minute presentation. Each member of the group makes a written choice of who gets their vote. Each candidate offers their views on their own performance. The group offers comments on the performance of the three candidates and what they were and were not impressed by. The teachers end the session after summarising the four elements of a successful election pitch:

1. Why is the candidate standing for this position?
2. What qualifications and experience does the person have that are relevant for this position?
3. What support does the person have for this role from other people and other groups?
4. What will the person do if elected?

CHAPTER 5

How to Prepare and Present a Poster for a Meeting

Preparing and presenting posters are skills that are often important for early career staff. How can you do this well? The skills discussed in this chapter are also related to the other chapters listed here.

Preparing the Poster

Posters may serve different purposes, for example, to present the results of a study during a scientific meeting, to inform people who come to visit an institution about previous work or about the structure of the institution, or to invite participants to join a programme or movement. In general terms, posters should not be used to present detailed reports about studies or about other matters, for example, the historical development of an institution. Regardless of its purpose, a poster must be easy to understand and remember. This imposes certain rules that should be observed in producing posters, namely:

- A poster should be *easy to read*. This means that it must have an *attractive title* and carefully prepared text no longer than one typewritten page (thus 32 lines).
- The poster should be printable (12-point font size) on an A4 sheet of paper and be easily *legible* in that form.
- The dimensions of the poster depend on the *instruction given by the organisers* of a congress (if the poster is prepared for a congress). Organisers of congresses usually have the dimensions of the poster announced on the invitation to the congress. When this is not done, it is useful to *contact the organisers* and ask what dimensions a poster should have. When this is not possible, we suggest dimensions of 70 × 120 centimetres (30 × 50 inches).

- The poster can *contain text or text and graphics*. The text of the poster must be *easily readable* from a distance of 2 metres. The same is true of the graphics, which should be understandable when viewed from 2 metres' distance.
- The *background* of the poster can be of a *pastel* colour. If an intensive colour is used, it is often necessary to increase the font of the letters and write them in a *contrasting colour*.
- If the text describes the results of a study, it should devote *at least one half of its space to the presentation of results* (if possible, in one or two illustrations).
- If the poster presents text, it should use *no more than three different colours* (e.g., black for the text, blue for the title, red for the main message). The text should be given with subheadings. For a description of a study, we suggest the following *space allocation*:
  - **An introduction** of two to three lines stating the problem and the answer (e.g., The high prevalence of mental disorders on the Istrian peninsula had no explanation until now. We have carried out a study that provides answers to this problem).
  - The description of the **methods** used (up to five lines).
  - The presentation of the **results** (using space of 15 lines).
  - The **discussion** (three to four lines).
  - The **conclusion** (two lines). It is often useful to place the conclusion as a subtitle for the poster.
  - One or two key references (three lines).

The poster *must be attractive*, and its attraction can be enhanced by using a photograph or a *graphically interesting* design. The photograph should not be frightening – photos evoking a pleasant feeling are more likely to attract viewers and be remembered. Graphic designs of posters can be helpful if they are *harmonious and pleasing*. It is useful to seek *opinions of colleagues* if the poster uses a novel and striking form. *Logos of the institution* in which the author works should be used if the institution and its logo are well known to the visitors to the poster.

It is useful to prepare an *A4 paper copy of the poster* and to have such copies available, possibly affixed to the poster stand in a large envelope, with a note ('Please help yourself to a copy of the poster'). The organisers usually provide the tools to affix the poster to the stand. It is, however, useful to take scissors, adhesive tape and tacks along. It is also useful to take some whitener, which will make it possible to correct any typing errors discovered just before the presentation of the poster. Finally, do be sure to include in large and legible text your name and contact details so that people who see and like your poster can contact you. See if you can include these people in your work networks.

Example of a Good Poster

We suggest that the poster shown below (Fig. 5.1) should be carefully studied as an example of an excellent poster. Published in 1809, this is the *Carte figurative des pertes successives en hommes de l'Armée Francais dans la campagne de Russe 1812–1813*

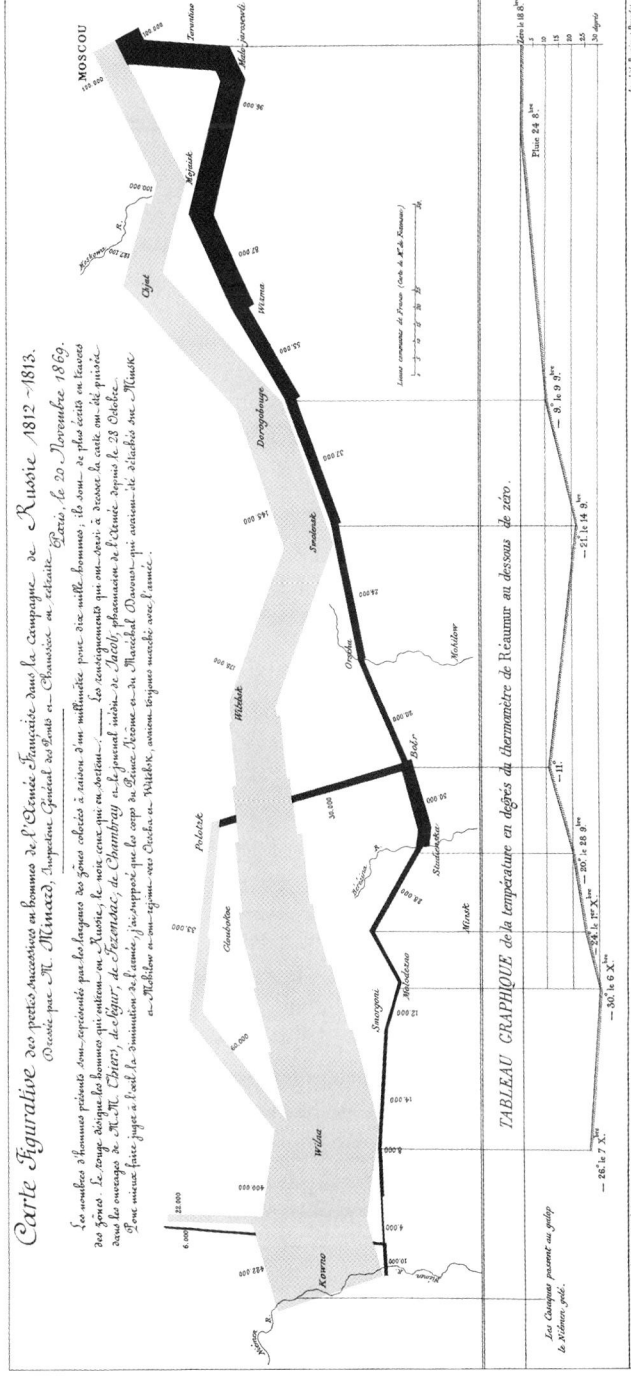

Fig. 5.1 Example of a good poster. (From Minard: Napoleon's Retreat From Moscow (Russian Campaign 1812–1813). https://masswerk.at/minard/)

by Charles-Joseph Minard. The poster shows the progress of **Napoleon's campaign** against Russia in 1812–1813. This image graphically illustrates that the army that began with 422,000 men was reduced to 100,000 when it was turned back at Moscow, and that only 10,000 soldiers survived on their return to France. The poster also portrays the temperature as a major factor in the war, and the locations of the main battles. Minard is credited with first inventing this type of 'flow map'.

Examples of Bad Posters

We suggest you put the following terms into a search engine or web browser: 'Example, bad poster, scientific conference, research', and then click on the 'images' option. You will find here many examples of truly terrible posters, which often share these characteristics:

- excess text and overcrowded visual appearance
- use of many colours in a way that is not attractive
- poor use of contrast of colours
- titles that are too long
- no clear statement of the names of the authors or their contact details
- too many visuals or graphics
- no clear logical flow to the presentation
- no clear presentation of the central message
- information that is hard to understand or retain
- nonstandard dimensions
- excessive use of citations or references

Many of the posters you can find on a simple web search will demonstrate many, if not all, of these characteristics of poor posters, from which you can learn.

Presenting the Poster

There are at least three ways to present posters.

1. In some situations, posters are displayed and the authors are not obliged to be in their vicinity. This way of presenting posters is becoming more popular, with an electronic presentation of the text of the poster that the visitor selects and then watches for as long as they please. This means that having prepared and submitted your poster to the meeting organiser, you have no other direct role except to respond to any queries that are sent to you by people interested in your poster.

2. In other instances the author of the poster stands next to the poster at a designated time or times and is available to answer questions that those visiting the poster area might ask. The time for which the authors have to be present is usually 2 hours, sometimes split into two 1-hour sessions.

3. Nowadays it is becoming usual to give the poster presenters a specific time when they must be next to the poster and then, during a 'poster walk', briefly

present their poster to the group that visits the posters in the area. The series of poster presentations in such situations lasts 1 or 2 hours and there is a chairperson who controls time and moderates the discussion. In this case, you may have just a few minutes to summarise your poster, and to try to engage your audience. We suggest that for this purpose you use many of the techniques we outline in Chapters 2 and 21 on how to make a presentation and to give an elevator pitch. Remember that you are selling yourself at least as much as the content of your poster.

When the posters are displayed and the authors are present next to their poster (option 2 discussed previously), you will need to respond to the requests and queries of visitors who ask for more information about a particular part of the poster. Or they may pose a more general question asking the author to describe the work presented in the poster – often referring to the specific sections of the poster (e.g., 'Did you have difficulties when applying your interview schedule to people of different cultural backgrounds?'). As the author of the poster, you should answer these questions as concisely as possible and try to engage the visitor in a conversation about the poster and its implications. Thus when asked about the scales used to assess attitudes, for example, the author should give a precise answer and continue with a question, for example, 'Is this questionnaire used in your country?' if the visitor is from another country, to start a discussion with the visitor and deepen the contact with the other person, and to explore if future collaboration may be possible.

In poster walks (option 3 discussed previously), posters are usually presented in rooms with background noise, with the speaker and listeners standing, and with a strict limitation to the time given to the speaker. This means that the introduction of the poster should be simple and sufficiently loud, focusing on the key essentials and avoiding too much detail. The presentation should start with a sentence or two summarising the main finding. After a brief pause, the presentation should continue with references to previous work in this field, starting with whether the findings confirm or contradict what others have previously found. The next few sentences should name the methods used (without describing them in detail – this can be done if the chairperson or a visitor asks for such information), and then refer to their validity and applicability. The speaker should not point to details of the findings shown on the poster, because that will mean that the visitors will watch the poster and pay less attention to the speaker. The presenter might end the presentation (which should last less than 2 minutes) by stating a problem for which the visitors might have a solution or might wish to advise, that is, by ending on an open or active question.

Please remember that the two chief goals of the presentation of a poster are (1) to present findings in a easily remembered form and (2) to identify individuals who have an interest in the matter and might wish to stay in touch with the presenter to continue discussion after the official presentation or possibly collaborate in the future.

In organised presentations (option 3) it is usually not possible to leave A4 printed copies of the poster next to it; therefore it is helpful to have a few copies available for you to give to your viewers who show an interest. It is also useful to have identified a place (e.g., a cafeteria or a stand) where it would be possible to meet people interested in collaboration should they wish to do so, after the poster walk is over.

The presentation of a poster can be considered a success if it results in links and possibly collaboration with others working on similar problems: a poster is an invitation to talk, to collaborate and build friendships.

Key Points

- The main ways to present a poster are (1) it is displayed when you are not present; (2) it is displayed when you are present for conference attendees to see; (3) it is displayed at a particular time when you are present, an organised group of people make a 'poster walk' and you have a short time to speak about your poster.
- If you can make a verbal summary be sure to give a brief summary; say if the findings of the poster confirm or contradict previous findings; mention plans for future work; and offer thanks to the chairperson and the listeners.
- The two main goals of the presentation of a poster are (1) to present findings in an easily remembered form, and (2) to identify individuals who have an interest in the matter and who might wish to stay in touch with the presenter and possibly collaborate in the future.
- The poster presentation is a success if it leads to a future collaboration or friendship.

Practical Exercise

Before the teaching meeting, each participant is simply asked to produce a poster. A session of the teaching meeting is set aside to discuss the posters. Each poster is discussed in turn. First the author is asked to summarise the poster in 60 seconds. The teacher then asks one or two in the group 'What is the main message of this poster?'. If the poster has not been well understood, ask the author to summarise the main message again, but more clearly than the first time. Comments are then invited from the whole group about what works better or less well in the poster. The teacher then offers specific comments on how to improve the poster, and will often stress that the poster should, first of all, clearly communicate its main, central message to the viewer. During the poster comments, stress the importance of rehearsal in preparing the poster and obtaining feedback before the formal presentation. As a variant for this session, use electronic rather than paper posters. This technique often requires the presenter to stand by the poster at a specific time and to give a 2-minute oral summary of the work. Stress the importance of knowing where the poster location is before the session, arriving early, rehearsing the oral presentation, and having your personal cards ready to give to poster session attendees to facilitate future networking. In practising the poster preparation and presentation, focus relentlessly on communicating the main message to the audience.

CHAPTER 6

How to Behave in an Interview With the Media

At any stage of your career you may have opportunities to work with the media to convey your point of view to large or very large audiences. We strongly suggest that you develop the skills to do this well. In our view, professionals have a duty to actively participate in public dialogue and debate about pressing issues of the day, and to do this with conviction, integrity and the public interest at heart. As in many of the other chapters of this book, we especially emphasise here the importance of *detailed preparation* before media interviews, in addition to honing your skills for the actual interviews, as well as for statements or talks you may be invited to give to the media. Related chapters are shown below.

RELATED CHAPTERS

Chapter 2. How to make a presentation or give a talk
Chapter 3. How to ask and answer a question at a meeting
Chapter 10. How to present oneself to a group of people
Chapter 12. How to prepare for a meeting
Chapter 15. How to write a report of a meeting
Chapter 18. How to behave in an interview for a post
Chapter 19. How to take part in a video meeting
Chapter 20. How to present a proposal for funding
Chapter 21. How to make an elevator pitch
Chapter 29. How to convince others about the usefulness of a project

Preparation for a Media Interview

Your approach to media interviews may be **proactive** or **reactive**. For **proactive media contacts**, you will first have to have a message to give to your intended audience. This could be about a new and promising service your team is starting to provide. Or you may be undertaking research and have exciting results that you are very keen to communicate. You can choose one or more channels or media to deliver your message. If this is the case, you would usually also prepare a *press release*. Typically, this would be a one-page summary of the core message comprising a brief background or context section; a slightly more detailed account of the core story;

and brief details of what will happen next or the implications of the story, followed by your contact details if any journalists wish to contact you.

What are the characteristics of an effective press release? It deals with important issues and gives clear data on the nature and the scale of the problem. It gives links for *further information*. In many press releases, the original website includes **graphics** (a map, as well as textual information). It cites **authoritative and verifiable sources** for the information. It gives **national and local** information. It also gives specific and *personal examples of individuals affected*.

Reactive media interviews refer to the situation in which a journalist or a media communications company or office contacts you, requesting an interview. In this case, we suggest that you **do not give the interview immediately** but find a time a little later on. Ask at the first contact the questions shown below, and then use the time before the interview to carefully prepare what you want to say. If you do not feel comfortable about the approach, for example, if the person who contacted you will not give you clear answers to your questions about the interview, consider not accepting the interview invitation. Although most journalists operate reasonably ethically much of the time, this is not always the case. In the field of mental health, for example, there is always the risk that people working in the media may report a story in an irresponsible or sensationalising way that increases stigma. If you are not sure that you can trust the journalist or company approaching you, then **be ready to quickly and gracefully decline the invitation** and say that you are unfortunately also unable to help them with their probable next question, namely who you suggest they can approach for an interview.

Questions to Ask if You Are Invited to Give a Media Interview

- Who would like to have an interview? Ask for the name and surname of the interviewer and if they working for a company (e.g., television, radio, newspaper, social media or podcast) or if are they freelance. Do they have a commission for this work or is it a speculative story?
- What is their time scale, i.e., when do they need to submit their copy or story?
- Why does the journalist want to cover this story now?
- What angle/approach will the journalist take for the story? For example, will they want to promote one side of a contested story, or invite you to take up an oppositional position in relation to another speaker, or portray you as exemplifying the 'medical model'?
- Who else is the journalist planning to interview?
- For broadcast news or features, or for print and online media, when will the story be made public?
- Is there any proposal that the journalist wants exclusivity, i.e., that you cannot speak with other journalists on this topic? If so, why, and with what embargo time and date?
- Will you have an opportunity to comment on the draft story?
- Will the journalist agree not to attribute to you direct quotes that you have not actually made?

- Is the request for an in-person, phone or video meeting?
- How long will the interview take?
- Who is the main audience for this interview, article or broadcast?
- For broadcast media, will it be prerecorded or live? On which station?
- If it is in person, will the media company pay for your travel costs to and from the studio?
- If necessary, tell the media person contacting you what you are prepared to be interviewed about and what you are not able to discuss.

If you do accept the invitation, the relentless news cycle often means that the journalist will want to speak to you quickly. If you have a busy day, try to *postpone some of your meetings to give you time to prepare well*. Try to find out *who will interview you*, and *who else may be interviewed*. What have they written or broadcast about recently? What is their work and educational background? Do they have any well-known or strong views on your topic or area of work? How *strong or weak is their reputation* in their field of the media? Of all the possibilities of how you can present your message, which version is most likely to *hook their interest*?

As in preparing a paper for presentation (see Chapter 2), the first and most difficult stage is to *decide exactly what you want to say*. Despite the temptation to include several messages in your communication, we strongly recommend that you focus entirely on *one central key message*. Very often this is not easy. Your clinical or research innovation may have several facets or components. You may have several startling or remarkable achievements or findings. But the likelihood that these will be picked up by the media reduces sharply if the number of central messages is more than one. You will also need to be acutely *aware of the current media environment*. This is a delicate balancing act as you will want your story to align with the *zeitgeist* or popular and fashionable issues of the time, without being derivative, dull or repetitive of other recent stories. Your message needs to be different from other similar recent news stories, but not that different.

Examples of Key Issues in the Current Media Environment

- Is there a **key topic** receiving extensive media attention, for example, the use of psychedelics for treatment?
- Is there a *scandal* that is hitting the headlines, for example, a recent series of suicides?
- Is there a *campaign group* that is having success in gaining media coverage, for example, for or against community mental health care?
- Is there a *client group* in the news a great deal, for example, military veterans with mental health conditions?

As you prepare your message for the media, you will see many similarities with how to prepare an ***elevator pitch***, which we discuss in Chapter 21, in terms of developing and refining a single, compelling and memorable message for your target audience. Keep in mind that you are likely to be speaking with a trained and ***experienced journalist***, and if they take up your story they are likely to want to answer most or all of the ***five W questions***: **who, what, where, when and why**. So prepare all these details in advance to save time. Also prepare a one-page summary of what you want them to pick up and publish and give them this just before or just after you meet. Try to find a short and striking, if not startling, way to compress your central message to grab the attention of the journalist. For example, compare the number of people who can be helped by your new treatment or research with a well-known quantity.

The central message needs of course to be ***honest and accurate***, but it should be presented in an ***eye-catching*** way, for example by drawing up a parallel with ***striking visual imagery***, such as the number of people in a full and famous football or athletics stadium, or the potential savings to be made by your innovation in relation to the average wage, or the total savings for the country as whole.

It is useful to find a friend, colleague or family member to try out your draft central message and ask if it does get your point across. Ask the person to whom you have spoken how the message can be made stronger or more immediate. ***Write down a small number of key points*** as abbreviated bullet points before you start your interview and keep these at hand to prompt you during the interview. Consider making your ***own video or audio recording*** of the interview if you are not sure how professional the journalist may be and in case you may want to have a full record or transcript of the interview at a later date.

How to Conduct Yourself During a Media Interview

Before the interview, make sure that the interviewer knows how to pronounce your name and has your correct job title and affiliation. At the start and during the interview, ***address your interviewer by name***. Maintain a positive and pleasant manner throughout the interview. Use a series of linking statements to make your key points, as shown below. Tend to use the ***bridging ABC technique***, as discussed in Chapter 3 on How to Ask and Answer a Question at a Meeting: acknowledge, bridge and communicate. People who are very experienced at dealing with the media can reply to virtually any question by getting their central point across. Whether the interview is for the broadcast, press or online media, it is likely that only a very small part of what you say will be picked up, if your interview is reported at all. Do not be shy about ***repeating your central message several times***. Use short words for this message. ***Avoid abstract or conceptual or jargon words***. If you want to make a general point, be sure to ***give a very specific example of what you mean***. Make your statements short. If the interviewer wants to attribute to you any comment that you have not made, or to put words into your mouth, firmly react against this, for example, by saying, 'Well Richard, in fact that is not what I meant, because the key point here is I…' and then give your main point briefly. Be ready to pause or give way if the interviewer wants to move to the next question or needs to bring the interview to a close.

Example of Poor and Good Practice in Conveying Your Key Point About Increasing Suicide Rates

- Do not say
  'You know I've always felt that somebody should be doing something about all the young people who die every year. The rates are very high you know, about as many as in car crashes, and there's always some background factor that should be understood, and I feel so sad when I hear about these events, and as a doctor I think each of these deaths could and should be prevented, and if I was the Minister of Health I would…' (is interrupted by the interviewer and the interview rapidly terminated).
- Do say
  'According to the WHO, around the world one person dies of suicide every 40 seconds. Every 40 seconds. This is a tragic waste of human life. But we do know what needs to be done. I urge the Minister of Health to take three steps immediately.
  One, to severely restrict the availability of pesticides. This works to reduce the suicide rates. Two, to ensure every school has a mental health counsellor. Young people need to access support at an early stage if they have mental health difficulties. Three, to ensure that painkillers such as paracetamol (acetaminophen) are only publicly available in blister packs. We estimate that 10% of all suicides can be stopped within 3 years in this country if these affordable and feasible steps are taken today.'

Do not become irritable, ironic, cynical, facetious or angry at any stage. *If you are interrupted* in a discourteous or unpleasant way, give way to the interviewer and as soon as you can continue and complete your previous point. *If you do not wish to comment* on a specific question or topic, especially if you have agreed in advance not to answer questions on a particular theme, give an immediate, short and flat reply such as 'I'm sorry but I can't help you with that'. Do not comment on what you do not want to comment about. Do not comment on issues outside your field of expertise. Be aware that the interviewer may be trying to encourage you to give a statement that directly contradicts what another interviewee will say. They may feel that *conflict sells*. Only engage in such a media conflict if you deliberately wish to do so. If you are invited onto a *phone-in radio show*, consider using the techniques that we discuss in Chapter 3 on How to Ask and Answer a Question at a Meeting.

Ways to Get Your Main Point Across

- 'Well I think the really important point here is to appreciate that…' (give your key point)
- 'My main message today, Tony or Sally, is that…' (give your key point)
- 'What I think most people are interested in is…' (give your key point)
- 'Despite what many people have heard, the fact of the matter is…' (give your key point)
- 'Before I come to your question, Tom or Jane, just let me say one thing…' (give your key point)

Debriefing After Media Interviews

If the interview was for the print or online media, follow up with that newspaper or outlet for several days to *see if your interview was included* in any story or feature. If the interview was for the broadcast media, similarly, check live or later online broadcasts to see if any of your interview was included or referred to. If you were covered in any way, pay careful attention to the difference between what you wanted to have picked up and included in the story, and what was actually included. Did the story accurately and fairly reflect what you actually said? If the report bears little resemblance to what you said, or directly contradicts your statements, ask yourself if you want to request a *right to reply* or to make a correction statement on social media. Ask friends and colleagues for feedback about whether the interview was successful in terms of conveying your main point to the intended audience. As recommended for many of the other chapters in this book, reflect on this experience, and analyse what went well or less well and *what you can learn* to make your next media interview even more brilliant!

Key Points

- If asked to give a media interview and you agree, do not agree to give the interview immediately
- Arrange a delay to give you time to prepare carefully and decide your single main message
- Do homework on the media company and the particular journalist
- Consider asking the key questions in the Questions to Ask if You Are Invited to Give a Media Interview features box above, before deciding to accept or decline the interview request
- As for other leadership skills, summarise the five W issues for your key points: who, what, where, when and why
- Use visual images or compelling analogues to convey your central message
- Express your central point in a way your key audience can quickly and easily understand

- Remain positive and courteous at all times during the interview
- Stay on your central message throughout the interview
- Use the ABC technique to link the question to the point you want to make
- Do not comment on issues outside your area of expertise
- Be cautious if you think you are being drawn into a conflict unless you chose to engage
- If the interviewer departs from preagreed topics or treats you with disrespect, be ready to stop the interview, and leave with a short and neutral statement of why you are leaving
- Debrief after the interview to see if you were reported at all, if you were reported accurately, and what you can learn to improve your next media interview

CHAPTER 7

How to Overcome Language Problems

This chapter discusses how to overcome language problems at work, and this topic relates to several other chapters as shown below.

RELATED CHAPTERS

Chapter 2. How to make a presentation or give a talk
Chapter 8. How to work with people from other cultures
Chapter 14. How to take part in a meeting
Chapter 19. How to take part in a video meeting
Chapter 31. How to work well in video and online collaborations

Regardless of how many words of a foreign language we know and how many books or articles in that language we read, most of us will – when speaking in a meeting or during an interview – occasionally **experience anxiety** and be unable to find the word expressing exactly what we would like to say. It is important to recognise that this is normal and expected, because if this is not done it can lead to at least three untoward outcomes:

- You may become reluctant to say something in a discussion because you feel that **you cannot say exactly** what you wish to say.
- You may make a special effort to **learn turns of phrase**, to a degree that will make the sense of your intervention lost in elegant constructions.
- You may present frequent and **unnecessary apologies** about problems that you experience in expressing yourself.

What to do about communication issues depends on the situations in which you find yourself. If you are in a social setting – having been invited to take coffee or a meal with people whose language is foreign to you – it is important to remember the following:

- Most people welcome someone who **listens carefully** to what they say, after all, listening is a sincere form of flattery and a tool to improve one's language skill.
- Think about things that you feel are important and **compose simple sentences** arguing for their acceptance. **Try them out** in a loud voice and if you have a friendly soul next to you ask them to tell you whether what you said was clear, convincing and interesting.

- Make your **interventions brief** and state them neither too loudly nor in a low voice – practising your pronunciation and tone can be useful.
- Be **generous with your smile**, and have a friendly and interested expression: if you do not feel friendly or interested leave with a polite excuse.
- Help those in whose company you are by **assisting them with their chores** – or at least offer help. People who like you and consider you helpful will be much more likely to listen to you and try to understand your position.
- The languages that people of the same profession, same age and same gender use are not the same, and they can **vary in their choice of words**, emphasis, loudness and use of technical terms. You might remember this principle when communicating with people with whom you share a mother tongue.
- Do not hesitate to **consult a dictionary** while thinking about a meeting or social event that you are going to attend. Think a bit in advance about the people who you will meet, and about topics that are likely to come up and which will be of interest to them.
- If people find the way in which you expressed your ideas amusing and have a friendly smile, **join them in their good humour** (rather than take offence).

Overall we suggest that language problems are **openly acknowledged** for meetings of people from different backgrounds and that people are ready to ask and to answer questions of one another to improve communication as much as possible. These suggestions are valid even if you speak the language of the people you meet very well, because they are not specific to difficulties of expressing oneself in another language, but rather can serve as a guide to improving social contacts with all the people you meet.

Key Points

- In a globalised world, it is common to work with people from other backgrounds and cultures, and who are using a language that is not their mother tongue
- Accept that all parties may need to show commitment and flexibility in communicating clearly with one another
- Try to make your own communication as clear as possible and do not use complex forms, such as irony or satire, that can confuse your true meaning
- Pay attention to positive and friendly forms of nonverbal communication
- Take time to work towards a clear and common understanding of what people from different language backgrounds want and need to communicate with one another

CHAPTER 8

How to Work With People From Other Cultures

Culture is a concept that has many definitions – someone counted them and found that there are over 50 – and what we call culture in this book refers to **culture as defined** as the values, habits and traditions of a group of people. This chapter is related to other chapters in this book as shown below.

RELATED CHAPTERS

- Chapter 7. How to overcome language problems
- Chapter 16. How to lead a small working group or collaboration
- Chapter 19. How to take part in a video meeting
- Chapter 22. How to negotiate
- Chapter 25. How to work in a small group
- Chapter 26. How to reduce tension in a small group or in a meeting
- Chapter 28. How to collaborate and use networks and feedback
- Chapter 31. How to work well in video and online collaborations

Working methods and patterns in modern times make it necessary to learn how to be, and how to work, with people belonging to cultures other than our own. When this is not done well, teams work poorly, misunderstanding of the intentions and actions of others is probable, and all those concerned – those in the 'home' culture and those in the 'other' culture – tend to be dissatisfied and nonproductive, often **blaming each other** for difficulties and failures.

All cultures have as their goal to improve the life of those who belong to it, often disregarding the harm that these improvements might cause to people in another culture. What most cultures tend to neglect is that the **similarities between cultures** are often much more prominent than their differences. Just what the differences are is often unclear, and the dominant tendency is to refuse to learn about them rather than to **try to understand** them. At best, other cultures and people who share them are considered unusual, not easy to understand and best avoided.

The first step to a satisfying collaboration or coexistence with people from other cultures is to **accept that they have the same rights** and same level of **obligations and duties** as everyone else. Next in importance is to **try to learn what rules and**

traditions characterise the 'other' culture and those who belong to it. Once this is clear, it is **important to give time** to agree on who does what and how.

It is also important to **seek ways of coexisting** with people from other cultures whom one meets or with whom one shares the same habitat, workplace or company. The basic rule in this effort is to understand that **one's own liberty of action must be defined by the rights of others** and that certain efforts must be reformulated because they are likely to harm those from a culture different from one's own. In a sense, a basic principle of getting on with people from other cultures is to start with the point of view of **respect for the other person**, just as one needs to start with respect for people from one's own culture. For example, if you make a mistake in introducing a person, such as mispronouncing their name, inappropriately offering to shake hands or inadvertently making a culturally unacceptable comment, this may be forgiven in the context of you having demonstrated that you respect the other person.

In practical terms, these guidelines mean that it is necessary to **reserve time for talking, exchanging information, and learning** about rules that govern the lives and actions of people from another culture. For example, before meeting people from another culture, make time to read about that culture and use some of these points as the basis for discussion when you meet, and to test if what you have read is in fact true now or not. Learning about the other's culture should not stop at learning about rules relevant to working together: the exchange of **information should cover traditions about the many ways of life and action regulated by culture**.

It is important to **jettison the idea that we know the basic rules that govern all people in all cultures**. Not only are cultures different: people who belong to them are different from one another and collaboration and coexistence depend on knowing enough about the other and on accepting the need to **find a mutually acceptable way of being and working together**.

We should keep in mind that our image and opinion about other cultures are often formed from **insufficient or wrong information**, that we must start from the position that we do not know much about the others' culture, and that it is necessary and useful to learn about it.

Furthermore, it is useful to remember that **people sharing a culture are also very different from one another**. It is therefore useful and necessary to **continue learning about other people**, their culture, their personality, and their wishes, intentions, strengths and weaknesses. This will make it easier to avoid conflict and improve the probability of **useful and productive collaboration**. It will also **diminish the probability of maintaining stereotypical ideas** about the preferences, strength and weaknesses of people from a different culture – prejudices that prevent the best use of the time, ability and skills of all.

Key Points

- The conditions of modern working life mean that it is vitally important to learn about the culture of other people
- Without such an ongoing effort, communication at work suffers, and a negative approach of blame can develop
- The similarities between cultures are often much more prominent than the differences
- Keep in mind that people from other cultures have the same rights and the same level of obligations and duties as people in your own culture
- One's own liberty of action must be defined by the rights of others
- Reserve time for talking, exchanging information, and learning about the rules that govern the lives and actions of people from another culture
- Accept the need to find a mutually acceptable way of being and working together
- People sharing a culture are also very different from one another
- Diminish the probability of maintaining stereotypical ideas of other people and other cultures

Skills Needed to Work Well in Smaller Groups of People

In the next section of this book we include short chapters about skills that will help you to work with smaller groups of people. For many people working in health or social care settings, work will often take place within clinical or practice teams. For this reason we cover several important aspects of team work here. We begin at the beginning as it is very often vital to introduce yourself to others and learn how to introduce others to a group. First impressions can have a lasting effect. Formal or informal meetings are likely to take up much of your time, and so we devote several chapters to how to prepare for, participate in and lead meetings, either in person or by video. Further important practical skills include how to prepare a job application and how to behave at a job interview. We go on to several more advanced issues that may be more relevant at a later stage of your career, such as how to deal with a poorly performing colleague, how to negotiate, and how to, kindly but clearly, say no. Many of these skills will also be helpful to you in talking to families or carers in your daily work, or to senior colleagues including governmental officials and health ministers.

CHAPTER 9

How to Introduce People at a Small Meeting

Introductions are important. How you remember others and how others remember you are strongly coloured by first impressions. This chapter gives you information on how to make a good first impression, both for yourself and for others. Other chapters related to this topic are shown below.

How to Introduce a Person to a Group of Similar Age and Professional Standing

Introducing someone is an opportunity to become known and remembered. You may be in a position to introduce another person to a group, for example, at the start of a teaching or professional meeting. We suggest that you have three goals in mind so that you introduce the person in a way that: (1) will make people recognise the person whom you are introducing; (2) will make you remembered as a nice person who is interested in others, and knowledgeable and respectful of the group and of your colleagues; and (3) will make the person whom you have introduced feel pleased by what you have said about them.

Preparing Your Introduction

Before making your introduction of the other person, talk to them, especially to **discover something unusual and memorable**. This might be the person's extraordinary knowledge about a subject, a skill (the best origami paper folder; the winner of the local cross country bike contest; fluency in the Coptic language) or some other unusual characteristic. If there is such a characteristic, ask the person whom you are introducing whether you may mention this in the introduction and, if so, include it in your introduction to **humanise the person**, and to make those present aware that they have the privilege of meeting someone who has a very special skill.

During your initial conversation with the person whom you will introduce, find out **how they pronounce their name**, and practice this to get it right. If it is complex, try to say it several times. If possible, use the person's original name and not an Anglicised name or version of their name. Most people are proud of their name and mispronouncing it can be hurtful and insulting.

If there is a personal detail that you would like to mention to the group when making the introduction (e.g., that the person is going to be married next week), ask the person whom you are introducing for **permission to mention** such a fact: in general, do not pass on personal details without that person's agreement.

Giving the Introduction

When your turn comes to make the introduction, **stand up** if you can, to give your voice stronger projection and to show your respect for the other person and the occasion. Even if you have made written notes about the person, do not look at these but rather remember the key points. Remember the rules about how to give a **short talk** (see Chapter 2): establish eye contact with each member of your audience; speak clearly and do not rush; and speak sufficiently (but not excessively) loudly. Smile and express pleasure about the fact that you will introduce the person. Depending on the occasion, aim to use a more formal rather than informal style, for example, by using a title such as Doctor if this is the case.

Your role is to pass on information to the group but, more importantly, to do so in a way that the group remembers, and has a **positive regard** for, the person you are introducing and wants to get to know the person more in the future. If you do the introduction well, that person will also have a positive view of you. If such introductions are done in pairs, that person is more likely to give a very positive introduction about you! To illustrate these key points, we include next examples of bad and good introductions for the following person: Dr Ivor de'Ath.

EXAMPLE OF A BAD INTRODUCTION

Speaking to the guest: I'm sorry, but what was your name again? OK, Dr Death. *Turning to the audience*: I will now introduce to you Dr Death. Ivor, if I may? Ivor is a very nice person, well known among his friends for his malicious gossip. He worked for a while in Asia, and then came back suddenly and unexpectedly to Europe. He has divorced twice but does keep in touch with some of his four children. He is a specialist in some transmissible diseases, and he worked in India for a while, with personal experiences of some of these conditions. We hope that he will resolve some of his interpersonal difficulties at work, and that the allegations against him will soon be shown to be without foundation. He can tell you himself about some of his many exotic hobbies. Without further ado I give you – Dr Death!

EXAMPLE OF A GOOD INTRODUCTION

I am delighted to introduce to you Dr de'Ath (pronounced 'day-ath'). He is an old school friend of mine and one of the greatest authorities on psychiatric problems related to malaria. He worked for the World Health Organization and for the British government as an expert in this field, and he has extensive real-world experience in several low- and middle-income countries. He has published a book, as well as numerous articles that are seen as classics. He is a man of great integrity and professionalism who continues in active clinical practice, alongside his busy research and teaching activities. The title of his talk this evening is 'Complex interactions between psychiatric morbidity and malaria'. Please join me in offering a very warm welcome to Dr de'Ath.

Key Points

- Your aims are to:
  - make people recognise the person whom you are introducing
  - remember you as a nice person interested in others, and knowledgeable and respectful of the group and of your colleagues
  - make the person whom you have introduced feel pleased by what you have said about them
- Discover something unusual and memorable about the person you are introducing, but include this in your introduction only with the person's permission
- Make sure you pronounce the person's name correctly
- Recall the rules about giving a short talk (Chapter 2) as you make your introduction
- Try to leave the group wanting to get to know the person you have introduced better

Practical Exercise

A good way to help people to introduce others is to arrange the group in an approximate circle and ask each person to introduce their neighbour to their immediate left. First, allow the group members 5 minutes to interview their neighbour. Then each participant introduces the person sitting to their left. Normally each introduction should be no longer than a minute or two. The introductions are made by going around the circle. The whole group is then asked what they particularly liked and disliked from the introductions, guided by questions from the teacher such as: Was it helpful when some people who made their introduction stood up. Why was this helpful? Which were the most memorable introductions and why? Was it relevant to say that the person is married or not? Was it helpful to mention the person's background experience in relation to the current meeting? This will help both the person making the introduction and the person being introduced to know what to say to others to help them make introductions. Participants also learn from hearing a series of introductions. The teacher can comment on particularly good or to less strong examples of introductions. When participating in a symposium, it is helpful for each speaker to give the chair a brief note to help that person to make the introduction in a brief and accurate way.

CHAPTER 10

How to Present Oneself to a Group of People

Making a good impression on others is an important part of building and enhancing your career. This chapter provides some guidance on how to do this well. Other relevant chapters are shown below.

RELATED CHAPTERS

Learn About the Group to Which You Will Introduce Yourself

If you learn that you will have to present yourself to a group of people, try to find out what the group is like. Is it hierarchical with some kind of ruler or chief, or a collegial group without a hierarchy? If the group is hierarchical, greet the group leader first and then look at the other members. Also try to learn whether the group pursues some topics with a great deal of emotional investment or whether it has no particular emotional commitment. Try to find out whether the group is in a particular mood, for example, if they have just experienced a loss, or perhaps won a prize. **Adjust your style to match the mood of the group**.

Dress and Behaviour

You should **dress neutrally** – neither too elegantly nor too shabbily, neither in strong colours nor in drab tones. Try to have a friendly and interested facial expression. Do not put your hands in your pockets, and if you are uncertain what to do with them take some object – a book, for example, or a pen, and hold it with both hands.

Contributing to a Discussion

You may be invited to join a group for a particular reason, for example, to bring your expertise to a specific discussion. We suggest the following:

- **Do not start speaking without an invitation** to speak, which will probably done by a person of authority in the group
- **Do not stare** at the members of the group
- But **do not look away** to the ceiling, floor or window; let your eyes, possibly with a friendly facial expression, sweep slowly along all those present, with short, nonaggressive eye contact with as many of the members of the group as possible without turning your head all the way to left or right.

Once you are invited to speak, if you have not been announced or addressed by name, briefly **say who you are**, pronouncing your name slowly and clearly. In some instances, if the group is relatively informal you might wish to make a comment about your name, e.g., if in your language it has a meaning (a profession [e.g., a tailor or a smith], a concept of nature [e.g., a geographical area or flower] or a personality feature [e.g., courageous]), to introduce a light tone or a note of humour from the outset.

If the group is formal, then pronounce your name clearly and do not continue to speak until you are asked to do so by the chairperson or someone who is asking questions. A slight bow in the direction of the chairperson is often useful to **show respect** to the person and to the occasion.

Try to assess whether the group that you are addressing has an **opinion on your professional or personal identity**. If they do, for example, if the group is composed of people who do not like or trust doctors in general or psychiatrists in particular, then you may wish to start by saying that you are aware of their opinion, but nevertheless you would ask members of the group to consider the information that you are presenting with an open mind.

Speak freely, **maintaining eye contact** with the members of the group unless you have to refer verbatim to some specific piece of text where the detail is important. If you fear that you might not remember all the points that should be addressed, shorten your list of key points. If you cannot remember your main points, the group members will certainly also have the same difficulty.

Do not forget to **thank the group** for listening to you, but do not end by saying that you will be pleased to answer questions. This is for the chairperson to decide and they will indicate if questions can be asked following your contribution.

Key Points

A presentation of oneself includes three components to keep in mind:
1. What the group will think of your appearance
2. What the group thinks of other people like you, e.g., other doctors
3. What you will say and how clearly and respectfully you express yourself

Practical Exercise: The Triplet

The whole teaching group is divided into small groups of three people. In each small group one person introduces themselves briefly for 2–3 minutes to the second person, while the third person observes this interchange. After this, all three offer feedback to each other on the introduction that was made. In step two, the roles are changed and the process is repeated. In step three the roles change again, also followed by mutual feedback, so that each person has the chance to (1) introduce himself or herself, (2) receive the introduction, and (3) observe the interaction. This technique can also be used for a range of other skills discussed in this book, for example, how make an elevator pitch.

CHAPTER 11

How to Chair a Meeting

An important leadership skill is to be able to chair a meeting well. This chapter sets out our views on what constitutes good practice in chairing meetings. The chapter refers mostly to in-person meetings. Other related chapters are shown below.

RELATED CHAPTERS

The Roles of a Chairperson of a Meeting

By 'chairperson' in this chapter we refer to the person who leads, coordinates and manages a single meeting or a series of meetings, and we sometimes abbreviate 'chairperson' to 'chair'. The role of chair has several closely related responsibilities. This person will need to convey the **purpose of the meeting to the participants** and seek agreement, openly or tacitly, on this purpose from the members of the meeting. The chair will need to **set the agenda** for the meeting and make it known to the members, preferably at least a week ahead of the meeting date. The chair will need to preside at the meeting to try to successfully **complete the business** of the meeting in the time available. Even if the business is important or serious, the chair may also try to ensure that the meeting is rewarding or even enjoyable for participants.

Another document that should be prepared if the meeting is not a routine meeting of a group that meets on frequent occasions is a **list of participants**, giving their name and position, which may be relevant to the decision making (e.g., advisor, head of a department concerned with the discussion, etc.). The list of participants should include all those concerned: if an invited person cannot attend, this should be marked on the list of participants.

Preparation for the Meeting

Perhaps the most important issue in preparing for a meeting is to **set the agenda**. Although the chair usually leads in setting the agenda, there are some occasions for which other senior staff set the agenda, and then the role of the chair is to moderate the meeting in which the agenda is discussed. We suggest that the items for the agenda are **numbered** and that an approximate **time allocation** is made for each item. Usually issues to be discussed at business or team meetings can be described as: (1) **for information** (e.g., announcing a forthcoming event or holiday); (2) **for discussion** (where the meeting members are invited to express their views on a topic); or (3) **for decision**. Some agenda items may combine more than one of these categories. It is usual to put the more **important issues higher up on the agenda**, especially where decisions are needed, so that there is likely to be sufficient time. Less important issues that are lower on the agenda can be discussed briefly or deferred to a later meeting.

Decide on the **information that needs to be sent** out to the members before the meeting starts. It is often useful to develop working papers presenting the facts and issues that should be discussed. Such working papers should be distributed with the agenda, if possible in advance of the meeting. A working paper is different from information about the background and materials that relate to it. Large volumes of information are less likely to be read, but for important decisions be sure to send out all the relevant material in advance so that members have this available to consider in detail if they can. Be sure to send out clear details of where and when the meeting will start and when it is expected to end. If there is a change of venue of a regular meeting, show this in bold and make a special note of this to committee members.

Preparing the Meeting Room

If you can control this, **select a room and a setting that will make it more likely for the meeting to be successful**. There needs to be enough room for members to not feel crowded, while also being able to hear each other very clearly. Is there distracting outside noise from lawn mowers or construction work? Can you control the room temperature? Do you have all the audio-visual aids you need? Will drinks or snacks be necessary? Can the members all see one another during the meeting? Who will be nominated to make a note or a record of the meeting? Are any fire alarms planned? Do you need to tell members what to do if there is a real fire alarm? Where are the toilets? Do you need to adjust curtains or blinds if there is strong sunlight? Is there good ventilation in the room? Is air conditioning noisy and can this be reduced? Do you need any aids such as a whiteboard or flipboards? Are there pens? Is the projector working and do you know how to switch it on, and is the remote control available and working? If you will use a computer in the room, will it work directly or do you need a password? Do you have contact details for audio-visual staff if you need help? Do you need a laser pointer?

Where to Sit as Chair of the Meeting

It is important to arrange the seating around the table in a manner that will allow the **chairperson to see all participants**. When the table is round this is easy; when the table is quadrangular it is important to think of ways to ensure non-verbal communication with participants. The chairperson may, for example, invite those participants whose face the chair does not see to comment or state their views. In rooms with lighting from the windows, the chairperson should neither have the windows behind them nor facing them because in both instances they will not see the facial expressions of the participants nor notice that they would like to speak. The chairperson should also not be sitting with their back to a door through which people might arrive during the meeting, because it will distract them, and possibly make it difficult to lead the meeting efficiently. For example, in Fig. 11.1 we show 18 possible seating options for the chair of the meeting, considering the shape of the table, the light from the window and the location of the door to the room. We suggest you consider, as chair of the meeting, sitting at a shorter end of the table to better allow you to see all the members of the meeting. The chair should not sit with his or her back to the door, because this makes it more difficult to be fully in control of the meeting when people or noises may enter the room from behind the chair's back. We suggest that the chair does not sit with their back to the window because this will give a silhouette effect for most people at the meeting and make it more difficult from them to detect nonverbal signals of communication from the chair, especially those on the opposite side of the table. For these reasons we suggest that the chair sits in position 17. In this

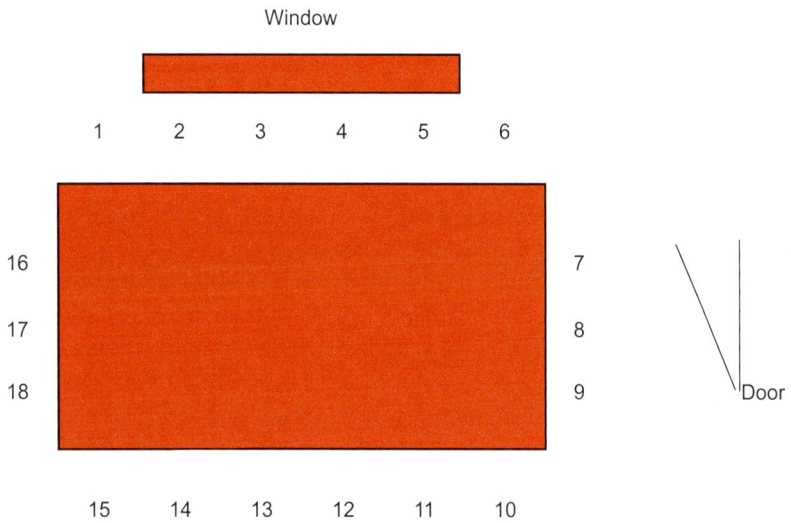

Fig. 11.1   Choosing where to sit as chair of a meeting.

case, we suggest that the secretary of the meeting sits immediately to one side, for example, in position 16. Keep position 18 for the most important person at the meeting, who may well need to leave the meeting after a brief introductory word. The person who will write the report of the meeting (the rapporteur) can sit, for example, in position 6.

Starting the Meeting

Arrive early. **Identify your seat** and occupy that place, for example, with your bag. Get up and pleasantly **greet each member** of the meeting as they arrive and try to make a positive personal remark. If you want any member to sit in a particular place, make this clear. **Start the meeting on time**. Check if the people present know each other. Allow a little time for **brief introductions** before the main business starts. Tell the members the time by which the meeting is expected to end. Some people may need to stretch and walk about, check email or messages, or to go to the toilet, so if the meeting is planned for more than an hour, **say if there will be break**, for example, for 5 to 10 minutes, during the meeting.

When opening the meeting and after the introductions of those present have been done, the chairperson should ask members to **look at the agenda**. The chair should the give an overall summary of what is on the agenda and say what they think are the **most important items**. It is usual for the first item on the agenda to be 'apologies' from members who are not able to attend. But we tend to favour **starting the meeting on a more positive note**, for example, by noting relevant items of good news, successes or achievements since the previous meeting. Ask if anyone cannot stay until the end of the meeting and see if you may need to reorganise the agenda to allow for this.

Moving Through the Agenda

Shape the discussion by telling the group if you have, for example, just 5 minutes remaining for the current item. Overall, tell the group if you see the discussion running over time and if you want comments to be more brief for the remainder of the meeting. If you are making faster progress with the agenda than you expected, then offer the promise of an **early finish** if this excellent pace continues. As you begin to finish each item on the agenda, ask yourself if you need to make either a summary statement of what has been discussed or decided upon, or, at an earlier stage, if you need to make a **provisional summary**, which you can then ask the group members to comment on. If there is agreement, you can go on to give your **final summing up** on each issue. If **disagreement** follows your provisional summary, you need to decide whether you think more time would help to resolve the issue, or if it may need to be deferred to a later meeting or managed in some other way, for example, delegated to a subgroup of the meeting.

When you want to **move to the next item** on the agenda, say clearly that you are about to finish the current item and ask for any other brief comments from group members. After you have closed that item, try **not to go back** to previous items on the agenda. As you start each new item, remind the group whether it is for information, discussion or decision. If an **item is for decision**, identify the specific issues that need to be decided. It may be helpful for you to set out a **series of options** for what you see as acceptable decisions for each item. If a proposal is made that you do not consider to be possible or desirable, say this immediately and say why.

If there are several breaks during the meeting, it is helpful for the chair to carefully observe who is speaking with whom and how warmly or cordially, and to identify **patterns of friends or colleagues** who can be expected to support each other during the formal parts of the meeting. Note as well which members of the group do not seem to be talking to others and appear to be **isolated from the group**. These observations will allow the chair to form a type of mental picture of the group in the form of a **sociogram**.

Do not allow the discussion to wander away from the agenda. If necessary, intervene early if **digressions** begin, and gently remind the group what is being discussed now. Try not to allow any members of the group to **talk too much**. If some **members are quiet** or silent, invite them to comment either by name, or more generally invite those who have not yet said much to offer their point of view. Assume that everyone present can make a useful contribution to the meeting if allowed or encouraged to do so. If **tensions begin to rise**, or there are open disagreements that begin to become angry, personal or offensive, step in immediately. You can take a break in the meeting, introduce a note of self-deprecatory **humour**, ask clearly for respect in all the comments from members, or even end the meeting early. Do not allow unpleasant exchanges between members.

Ending the Meeting

Try very hard to **finish the meeting on time** or ahead of time. Be courteous and gracious in thanking members for attending and in showing that you value their time. Decide if you want to allow any discussion of '**any other business**'. In general, having the item 'Any other business' or 'Miscellanea' puts the chairperson into a position of having to deal with matters for which they are not prepared, and we advise not to have such an item on the agenda. Clearly summarise the **actions that have been agreed** at the meeting. Signal the date, time and place of any **next meeting**. Say when the meeting has ended. **Do not allow false endings** of the meeting when some members raise further issues or try to revisit earlier discussions, after you have closed the meeting. For more formal meetings make sure that it is clear who will produce the **draft minutes** or record of the meeting, and check this carefully before it is sent out to members. After the meeting, ask a few trusted colleagues for **feedback** on how you chaired the meeting and what you could do better next time. Reflect on their comments.

Key Points

- The preparation phase is critical for a successful meeting
- Usually the chairperson will need to set the agenda and often needs to send out papers for the meeting well in advance, for example, a week before the date
- Decide if each item on the agenda is for information, discussion or decision
- Prepare the room and audio-visual materials carefully to encourage a successful meeting
- Arrive early and greet group members individually
- Start on time
- Arrange for introductions of group members
- Indicate at the start of the meeting which items on the agenda are most important
- Allocate most meeting time to the most important items, and keep forward momentum
- Use humour to diffuse any tensions at the meeting
- Before finishing the meeting, summarise the main discussion points, decisions and actions
- End on time

Practical Exercise

A HOSPITAL MANAGEMENT COMMITTEE MEETING

Timing

The role play will require approximately 45 minutes (or less if the discussion runs out of steam or if the chair completely loses control of the agenda) and the discussion that follows may take a further 30 minutes.

Participants

The role play requires the active role play involvement of seven participants. The roles that should be assigned by the teachers to the players are:

1. The **chairperson of the hospital management committee**. The chairperson should be a participant who is not very assertive, is kind to all, and possibly not particularly good at planning and debating. The chairperson is relatively new to the hospital, is not given instructions about how to run the meeting, and does not know very much about the participants.

2. **Head of department 1**. This participant has a specific proposal for the expansion of their own department and will be saying why this proposal is being made.

3. **Head of department 2**. This participant has already prepared a competing proposal, which they do not disclose. Their main goal during the meeting is to block every proposal made by any other committee member that may reduce the money available for new projects.

4. **Senior administrative officer.** This participant brags about their connections with powerful people, about being able to provide funds, and about their links with power. They misbehave during the meeting, for example, they take calls said to be from the Minister of Health, walking out and returning to the room. They interrupts others and pay little attention to the chairperson.

5. **Person with a mild hearing deficit.** This participant does not want others to know that they have a hearing deficit. They make somewhat irrelevant comments, and often ask that proposals be repeated.

6. **Person who is in a hurry.** This participant does not say they are in a hurry, but keeps hurrying the meeting along, interrupting discussions by asking the chair to make decisions, although the discussion has not yet been completed.

7. **Obsessional person.** This participant wants every issue to be very clear and specified in great and irrelevant detail (for example, asking what type of filling will be used for sandwiches), and often repeats what has been said to confirm that they have fully understood the discussion or the conclusion.

Format

The agenda is made available to all the participants, except to the person in a hurry. The role play is performed by the participants sitting in a circle or a semicircle, so that other students can see them from a medium distance (e.g., 5 metres away). Note that in the example shown below of a committee meeting agenda, each item is shown as for information, discussion or decision and with an indicative time shown for the duration of each item.

Meeting Agenda

12ᵗʰ Meeting of the Management Committee of Chub Hospital
Draft agenda

Item	Topic	Purpose of the item	Duration (minutes)
1	Welcome and opening remarks	Information	5
2	Planning the farewell party for Chief Nurse Essenmoler	Discussion and decision	30
3	Request by the Hospital Director to prepare a list of publications produced by staff of each of the hospital departments	Information	5
4	Use of funds offered by the City government to the hospital	Decision	15
5	Introduction of two new staff members	Information	4
6	Date of the next meeting	Information	1

Debrief

After approximately 45 minutes of discussion, the chairperson will close the meeting (with the meeting length to be agreed in advance). In the debrief, the members of the committee are each asked to describe their experiences of the meeting, to guess why the participants behaved in the way they did, and to comment on their experience of the committee. The teacher specifically asks the chairperson to guess why the members of the committee were behaving in the way in which they did. The other participants in the role play should also be invited to say what they have seen, and also to comment on each of the committee members. After this, the observing students on the course are invited to make comments and ask questions. A general discussion will follow.

Key Points for General Discussion

These should include the following:

1. The need to control persons behaving in the manner of participant 4. The usual method is to load them with tasks, which often results in their absence from the next session of the committee.
2. The chairperson needs to speak with all the members of the group before the meeting, which will help in running the meeting knowing the needs and intentions of the members.
3. People with obsessional tendencies may be very useful as note takers.
4. The chairperson should establish whether anyone needs to leave before the end of the meeting, which will reduce the nuisance of one member hurrying the meeting along.
5. A person with impaired hearing might be helped by having them sit next to the chairperson, who can also regularly summarise the state of the discussion for the benefit of the person who does not hear well. The chair can also suggest to the person to meet afterwards and go through the main conclusions of the meeting together.
6. Before the meeting, the chairperson should have talked with the two department heads to establish how best to handle their competition, thus preventing a fight during the meeting.

The role play usually offers triggers for the discussion of other issues and observations that might arise in departmental and other meetings, as set out in Chapter 13.

CHAPTER 12

How to Prepare for a Meeting

Meetings may be a very important part of your work. In other chapters of this book we discuss important aspects of meetings, including how to chair, introduce participants, take part in in-person and video meetings, and write meeting reports. This chapter aims to help you to **prepare for a meeting**. Related chapters are shown below.

RELATED CHAPTERS

Chapter 11. How to chair a meeting
Chapter 14. How to take part in a meeting
Chapter 15. How to write a report of a meeting
Chapter 19. How to take part in a video meeting

Before the Day of the Meeting

When you receive information about a future meeting, first of all **decide if you will take part** or not. Taking part can mean attending in-person, attending by video or other remote means, or attending some or all of the meeting. You can also contribute to a meeting by sending **advance comments** on some of the meeting items, for example, if you cannot attend the meeting itself. If you choose to attend only part of the meeting, decide which items on the agenda are most important to you, and mention to the meeting chair, before the meeting starts, if you need to arrive late, or leave early (or both!). If you cannot stay for all the meeting it is courteous to give the chair a reason for this. Before deciding whether to attend the meeting at all, ask yourself '*Why* **should I attend** this meeting?'. Consider the other good uses you could make of this time. If you have more than one meeting planned for the same time, think carefully about whether to attend either one, or part of both, or neither. Perhaps also consider the different **reasons you may wish to attend a meeting**, for example, to learn about a subject, to be seen, to meet some people, to present something, to please the chairperson or those who invited you, to return a service or to fulfil a promise. On some occasions you will conclude that the reasons to attend outweigh the reasons not to attend. There may be situations in which you are not sure whether to spend your time attending a particular meeting or not. In this case, you could write a brief list of reasons to go or not to go, bearing in mind some of the issues shown below before making your decision.

Possible Reasons to Attend or Not to Attend a Meeting

Reasons to Attend

- To see someone you want to meet
- You are obliged to attend
- To return a debt
- To meet people whom you respect or need or both
- To obtain new information important for your work and future action
- To affect the course of action or of a project that will be discussed

Reasons Not to Attend

- The meeting is badly prepared
- The participants are unpleasant
- The probability of learning something new is low
- It is a formal meeting of no practical use to you
- An alternative meeting at the same time is more attractive to you

Identify the Purpose of the Meeting

To help you decide whether you will attend, or how much of a meeting you will attend, find out in advance what the **purpose of this particular meeting** is. If it is not clear, for example, from the agenda or meeting papers, you may need to ask other participants about what they see as the aim of the meeting, and to see if they agree. A **meeting with no written agenda**, or no clear purpose, may in fact be very important, but this could be a danger signal that only a subgroup of participants have heard informally about the real agenda. For a meeting with no written agenda, try to decide if this indicates that nothing of importance will be discussed, or whether issues of great importance will be covered, but without giving participants the chance to prepare for the discussions or decisions in advance.

Apart from the formal agenda, decide if **you have other goals** that you want to achieve that will make it useful for you to attend. For example, you may want to have an informal word with a person who is important in your organisation, to advance or to block a plan that is vital for you, either before or after the main meeting. Other informal reasons that might favour attending the meeting include general **networking** or specifically introducing yourself to influential colleagues, to **showcase** your skills or knowledge to people at the meeting, or to **observe the meeting participants** carefully to see if they stand for or against particular issues within your organisation. Another potential benefit is for you to analyse **how the meeting chair acts**, and to draw your own conclusions and lessons about good and bad practice in chairing meetings.

Brief Yourself Before the Meeting

If you decide to take part in the meeting, your effectiveness is to a large extent dependent on how well you **prepare by briefing yourself** for the meeting. Read the **Terms of Reference** if these are available, to understand this framework for the event. Learn who is expected to attend and their respective roles. For meetings that are very important to you, try to get past minutes, for example, for all the meetings in the last year, so you can see the nature and pace of the discussions and what has been decided recently. See if the attendance for most meetings is strong or weak – weak attendance usually indicates meetings in which few important decisions are taken. Try to find out if this meeting has much **power or influence**. Know before you attend if you are there in a **personal capacity**, in which you can say more or less what you want, or if are you attending to **represent another group**. In the latter case, you may need to consult your group so you know what you are mandated to say, and also to feedback the details of the meeting to your group afterwards. Check to see if you have **any formal role** at the meeting, for example, to write minutes or a note of the meeting.

Before the meeting, **read the agenda carefully**. Focus on items for decision and make your mind up about whether you intend to speak **for or against specific proposals**. Prepare your comments and arguments in detail, possibly with written bullet points. Decide in advance if you will make any **counterproposals**. You may also want to discuss items with colleagues before the meeting to see if they **share your priorities or concerns**, and to coordinate your views.

Check the **time and place**. Regular meetings sometimes change their day, time or venue – it is embarrassing to arrive at the wrong time or to be in the wrong place. See if the meeting has both a start and a stop time. Decide in advance what you will do if the **meeting overruns** its allocated time. Be sure to know if the meeting is in-person, online or hybrid, and ask which option is better for you and better for the work of the meeting. If you will make preprepared comments on some of the agenda items, will you want to prepare slides? Will there be **audiovisual equipment** at the venue to allow you to use slides quickly? Do you need to arrive even earlier to pretest this?

See if the agenda allows '**Any other business**', and if there is something important you want to raise, tell this to the meeting chair, preferably before the meeting starts and saying how long you would like to have for this new item. Be aware that the chair may refuse to include your issue or only include it briefly. Prepare for your **travel time** to and from the meeting in relation to your other commitments on that day. If you have meetings directly before or after this specific meeting, check with the organisation administrator if they can provide you, for example, a **side room** for a separate earlier or later meeting.

On the Day

Arrive early and for large organisations, allow an extra 15 minutes, for example, to find your way to the meeting room after arriving at the main reception desk. Before the meeting starts, if you see people you do not know, consider approaching them to

introduce yourself and to find out who they are – the chair may or may not introduce meeting participants to each other at the start of the meeting.

Make time for a word with colleagues before the meeting starts, either for **informal and pleasant networking, or for specific issues** you want to raise quietly with particular colleagues. Think about who you would like to **sit next to** at the meeting and why. If this is important, place your papers or bag on your chosen place early on.

As you take your seat, complete your preparations before the meeting starts, for example, by plugging in the **charging cable** for your phone or laptop. For important meetings, be sure to bring a way to make an unobtrusive **note of the meeting**. Congratulations – you are now very well prepared, before the meeting starts, to make good use of this time.

Key Points

- First of all, decide if you will attend a particular meeting or not
- If not, you can send your comments on the agenda in advance to the chair
- Check to see if there is a clear purpose for the meeting
- Assess if attending the meeting will bring you or someone else a clear benefit
- Prepare yourself for the meeting well in advance. Read the relevant documents
- During the meeting, see what you can learn from the behaviour of others present
- See if you have any particular activity to undertake during the meeting or a formal role to play
- Notice the specific venue and time of the meeting – for regular meetings these can change
- Arrive early and take a more important seat at the table
- Consider what opportunities you can make or take to have informal meetings before and after the main meeting that can be of interest or advantage to you

CHAPTER 13

How to Chair a Conference Session

Taking part in conferences can be an **important part of developing your career**, especially if you work in the health service or at a university. It gives you the **chance to be visible** to people who can help you in the future, and to positively impress them. Other chapters (see below) discuss several aspects of taking part successfully in conferences. This chapter offers guidance on how to chair a session at a conference.

RELATED CHAPTERS

Chapter 2. How to make a presentation or give a talk
Chapter 3. How to ask and answer a question at a meeting
Chapter 5. How to prepare and present a poster for a meeting

Before the Session
BEFORE THE DAY OF THE SESSION

We offer the following advice having seen (or sometimes taken part in) all of the following preparations going wrong. First of all, do not accept an invitation to chair a session unless you are **knowledgeable about the subject matter** of the session topic. Look at the meeting programme well in advance and **check the time and place of your session**. It may not be in the main venue, and for some large conferences your session may be in a building a long distance away. Remind yourself what type of meeting it is, for example, a traditional-style session with a series of separate speakers, or a more modern-style meeting with speakers arrayed on sofas, about whom you are expected to make brief introductory remarks before they interact with one another in an informative and entertaining way.

Quite often a conference will arrange two session chairs, for example, in case one does not attend. If this is the case, try to **make contact with the other chair** before the session and plan who will do what, for example, who will open the meeting, who will introduce which speaker, and who will close. Check if you agree that you aim to start and stop the meeting punctually.

Visit the room or venue before your session, for example, the day before. Check the details of the podium, where you will sit, and the position of microphones, pointer and slide changers. See how you can change the light or lighting if you think it is too bright or too dark. Note if there is any distracting external noise and ask if this can be reduced. See if the seating layout is likely to contribute to a successful session, for example, by not having the audience sitting a long way from the speakers. Find out who the **audiovisual staff** are who will support the session, get their contact details and, if possible, make contact with them before the session in a friendly way – you may need to rely on them urgently if things go wrong. We also suggest you **visit the meeting venue the day before** you chair the session. Ask a friend or colleague to stand at the back of the room and give you feedback about whether they can see and hear you from the chairing position or table, and also check if the person standing at the podium delivering a talk can be seen and heard.

Get **brief biographies** for each of the speakers to help you to introduce them. Be sure to identify a strength or interesting positive characteristic for each speaker. Before you begin the session, **greet each speaker** and check that all are present. If any speaker is not there, tell the others about any change in the sequence of talks, and decide how you will use the extra time. For example, you can allocate longer to questions and answers. Ask each speaker **how to correctly pronounce their name**. Remind each speaker of just how little time they have for their presentation, and how you will remind them, for example, with comments at 2 minutes and 1 minute to go. Be fair to all speakers by making sure they **stick to their allocated time**, which mainly means **not letting early speakers talk for too long**.

Note also that if you are invited to moderate the discussion in a panel session where there is no specific allocation to titles and times of talks of the participants, it is useful to **write a synopsis**, in other words, a summary of how the meeting will run, who will be called on to speak first, second and so on, and what kind of questions you are likely to ask. Writing the synopsis will make it clear for you what will be happening – and you can also send the synopsis to the participants to orient them about your plan (and time allocations) for the session.

Decide before the session on how you **plan to use the time**. Will there be time for questions after each speaker, or at the end for questions for all speakers? For the latter, will you invite all the speakers to the stage? Are there enough seats on the stage? Is there another session in the venue immediately after your session so that you will need to finish and vacate the room on schedule? Know in advance if the session will be filmed or recorded and whether this is acceptable to the speakers. If it is a hybrid conference, make sure that the speakers are aware of this and who will be watching them. If they have any confidential material, for example, prepublication study results, discuss with the speakers whether they need to state any limitations to its wider dissemination.

On the Day of the Session

On the day, **arrive early** at the venue and check that key venue arrangements have not changed. Often rooms have changed their layout overnight or the laser pointer has disappeared. Just before your session starts, check that there is **water for each**

of the speakers, as many will be nervous and have 'dry mouth' syndrome. If **microphones** are used, check if these are static or mobile. Always **assume microphones are live** and that everything you say can be heard by others. If you are near a microphone, do not say anything that you would not like to see posted for the world to see or hear on social media a few moments later.

If you have not already met the audiovisual staff, try to find them, make a pleasant greeting and check for any difficulties from their point of view. Do the same with any **interpretation or translation staff**. Their level of cooperation can make or break your session.

As the audience begins to arrive in the room, consider whether to encourage them to sit near the front of the room to provide a more convivial, interactive atmosphere, or to allow them to huddle at the back of the room, with an empty and dispiriting area between speakers and audience. Do not worry if the audience is relatively small – it is their degree of interest and their contributions that will matter.

Before the session starts, **prepare in advance at least one question** to ask each speaker in case the audience is slow to engage with comments. If the format of the session is an interactive discussion between speakers sitting on sofas, give a clear structure to the speakers in advance. For example, for an hour session, allow each of four speakers to make opening remarks for 5 minutes on the session topic (without slides). This can be followed by a structured discussion of 20 minutes, led by the chair, on key headings related to the topic, encouraging active agreement or disagreement between members of the panel. Then have 15 minutes of questions and comments from the audience, with a 5-minute summing up at the end.

During the Session

THE PRESENTATIONS

Start on time. A late start takes time away from the session. Open by greeting the audience and giving the title (and sometimes the number) of the conference session. Some people may then realise they are at the wrong place or have the wrong time and quietly leave. **Create a positive tone** to the meeting by saying what an exciting topic it is and what great speakers are about to contribute. Tell the audience the structure of the meeting, namely how many speakers, and if there will be questions after each speaker or at the end of the session. Briefly introduce the first speaker. While they start, check that the slides are visible to the audience and that the audience can hear the speaker clearly. If the speaker is struggling to get the first slide ready, or use the slide changer or laser pointer, go to help them or ask the audiovisual staff to help.

Politely and clearly tell each speaker when their time is about to run out, for example, by giving them warnings at 2 minutes and 1 minute to go. If they reach their **time limit, firmly** ask them to sum up now.

Timing of Session Talks

Good practice example: Tell each speaker before the session what their time limit is and then keep to it

Bad practice example: Letting the early speakers exceed their time allocation and then asking later speakers to cut short their time

QUESTIONS AND ANSWERS

During question time, ask audience members to **raise their hand** if they would like to comment, or for a larger meeting, to come forward and line up behind the audience microphone. Tend to invite them to comment in the order in which they catch your attention. Allow them only one question each. Be sure to insist that all communications are **polite and respectful**. If a speaker seems not to have heard a question clearly, or may have misunderstood the question, the chair can help by paraphrasing the question for the speaker. If feelings rise, intervene to calm the spirits, for example, by reminding the participants of the limits of the topic to be discussed in this meeting, then move to the next person with a question. **Shape expectations**, for example, by saying 'I'm afraid we only have time for one more question'. Encourage audience members to make contact with speakers after the session closes, if time runs out. If a question is unclear, ask the person to paraphrase their point. If the question is not audible to the speaker or if they seem to be struggling to know what to say, help them by **restating the question** rather slowly to give the speaker more time to gather their thoughts. If there are no immediate questions for a speaker, give the group, for example, 10–15 seconds to allow contributions, and then use your preprepared question for that speaker.

CLOSING THE MEETING

As you close the meeting, **thank the speakers** for their excellent talks and the audience for taking part in the session. Try to create an atmosphere so that all can feel they have enjoyed the session. Actively suggest that people can **contact each other** after the session. If there are any subsequent related conference sessions, mention this. Be sure to make **the end of the session clear and formal** so that people know when they can leave. Do not allow further comments for the whole group after you have closed the meeting. If there is another session in the same room that starts immediately, suggest that your participants leave the room straight away and continue discussions outside.

After the Session

Thank each speaker individually at the time, and possibly also with a follow-up email, and say how much you enjoyed what they had to say. **Thank the other chair**. **Thank the audiovisual and interpreting staff**. Find a quiet corner for a strong cup of tea or coffee and relax for a moment before your next conference session.

Key Points

- Prepare carefully for the venue, the speakers and the conference support staff
- Make the cautious assumption that anything that can go wrong will go wrong
- Produce a synopsis of the session and share it with the speakers beforehand
- If you are chairing a panel session, write a brief summary, including reasons for having the session, the main issues to be addressed and the things that should not be part of the panel discussion. Be sure to know how to pronounce each speaker's name correctly
- Be flexible in case some speakers, or another chair, do not attend
- Start on time, keep each speaker to time, and end on time
- Create a positive atmosphere so that everyone is likely to enjoy the session

CHAPTER 14

How to Take Part in a Meeting

This is part of a series of chapters on how to make the best use of the time you spend in meetings. In this chapter we focus on what to do during a meeting. Related chapters are shown below.

The Start of the Meeting

Try to make **eye contact** with everyone present, unless it is a very large meeting. If you have not already greeted a person before the meeting starts, see if you can offer a **kind, nonverbal** signal or glance to indicate that you approach the meeting in a pleasant and nonconfrontational way. In particular, try to greet somehow **people whom you have not met before** – they are **potential future allies** for you. As the chair starts the meeting, look at your papers to **remind yourself of the agenda** and which issues will be most important to you. Arrange your papers if you need to have your notes ready for a preprepared comment. If you need to **fetch a drink**, do this before the meetings starts. Unless you have some urgent matter external to the meeting, **switch off your phone** or turn down the volume. If there is loud noise outside, or if the room is far too hot or cold, ask the chair if you can help by changing this.

The Body of the Meeting

For medium to large meetings, for example, up to 50 people, try to **look interested** in the topics of discussion, even if you do not find all of them riveting. It is discouraging for a meeting chair to look around the table and see bored faces. See if the culture of the meeting suggests that participants can carry on with other tasks such as **checking email**. If in doubt, err on the side of caution and show respect for the occasion by **not multitasking**. If you are **feeling critical** of how the chair is behaving, for example, allowing lengthy discussion about trivial items, try not to show this or make any critical comments. Sooner or later you will want the chair to favour you in some way, so try to be friends with them.

Try to **time your comments** carefully. If you have strong views about a particular issue that is discussed, decide if you want to make your opinion clear to others early on when that item is opened, or whether to wait until you have a more detailed sense of the views of others, before you decide how strongly to express yourself. If the meeting is to last a longer time – say, have three or four sessions – you might wish to speak to people about the proposals that you are going to make or your objections to something that has been presented, and ask for their comments before you present them formally. When the chair is trying to close an item and tries to make a **summary statement**, decide if this is a fair summary of what has been said, and in particular note if this summary has paid enough attention to any comments you made. If not, remind the chair of your point of view if you want this to be formally noted. Do not make this comment by saying 'Chair, I must draw your attention to the fact that the proposal (or comment) I made is not recorded in the minutes of the meeting'. Rather, ask in which part of the report it might be best to include the proposals that you presented.

Note, as the meeting goes ahead, **how people are behaving**. If participants want to make a comment, do they simply speak when they wish, or do they indicate to the chair, for example, by raising a hand, that they are **ready to comment**? Judge how polite and managed or unmoderated or even aggressive the discussion is, and then decide if you will take part on the same terms, or if you will be more or less assertive than most of the others present. If you do raise your hand and are not invited to speak, you will probably want to try again until the floor is yours. Try to make your **comments brief** and to the point, unless you feel strongly that you need to make a more detailed or a more impassioned comment at a key moment before a decision is made. On most occasions you will have just as much right as any other person at the meeting to offer your opinion in as much detail as you wish.

If you **agree with a point** made during the meeting, do make a **positive comment** to say you agree or strongly agree with what was said. People making a comment usually very much welcome others who support them. You may also go on to give further reasons why a particular proposal is a good idea. As you do this, look around the room for **nonverbal signals** of agreement, disagreement, neutrality or boredom, to gauge the sentiment and balance of feeling of the group on that specific issue.

If you disagree with a point made by another participant, you may need to say this clearly and politely. It is usually more constructive not to criticise a person for their comment, but to **'depersonalise' the issue** and disagree with a point raised, while at the same time making your respect for the other person clear, directly or indirectly. For example, you might acknowledge that the other person has raised an important point, and then go on to say 'Here's another way to look at this issue', before you offer your perspective. It is usually a mistake to show anger during a meeting, even if others are doing so.

Try to end each meeting with **relationships with others intact** and on at least a neutral basis, even if you have had to disagree with them on some specific issues. You are very likely to need to discuss other issues with group members at a later date and lingering negative feelings will not help you to achieve **your future goals**.

Try not to **interrupt** another person while they are speaking and if you do so unintentionally, apologise. If someone else interrupts you, look to the chair for assistance. If none is forthcoming to help you, it is usually better not to speak at the same time as the interrupter, but to wait for them to finish and then for you to restart your comments calmly at the point where you were interrupted.

Often there are points in a meeting when an action is suggested and the chair looks forlornly around the meeting for someone to **volunteer to take on the task**. The proposal for the action is commonly made by someone who has no intention of actually taking on this task. Pause before committing yourself and assess if you really want to accept this role. Do you have the skills, time and resources to do it well? Would it interfere with **more important work** that you have already committed to? If you are asked directly to take on a task, unless you are immediately sure that you want to do this, either **gracefully decline** or broadly mention that you are happy to consider the issue, but that you cannot make a commitment without carefully considering the matter. Try to avoid leaving meetings with an increasingly long list of tasks you have committed to in the weary knowledge that you will never be able to do many or most of them.

The approach needed for a relatively short meeting, for example, an hour or two long, may well be different from a longer or more complex meeting. For example, it is common for a large project or programme of work to have a **long annual meeting**, which can take 2 or 3 days. This may be to review progress since the previous meeting for the components of the programme; to address as a whole group difficult or controversial topics; to engage with important members of stakeholder groups; and to plan ahead for the work that needs to be done before the next large programme meeting. For these larger meetings it will often be necessary to have a clearly planned and timetabled agenda, to make best use of the scarce time the group has together, and to identify in advance which important decisions need to be taken at the meeting. We also suggest that such in-person meetings clearly include time to build, maintain and enrich the relationships between colleagues and collaborators, to give importance to the **relational, as well as the transactional, elements** of the working group.

The End of the Meeting

If you need to leave the meeting before it has finished, try to **catch the eye of the chair** to indicate that you are sorry to need to go, and leave quietly. Ideally, you should alert the chairperson that you will have to leave at a certain time. Do this by speaking to the chairperson beforehand, not during the meeting. When the meeting does end, decide if you want to stay a little longer, to chat to new or key people, or to **debrief on the meeting** with colleagues or allies, and build that time into your diary. If the chair managed the meeting well, offer a sincere **word of congratulation** on a meeting well led. If the meeting was not well chaired, do not comment. To support networking, have your paper or electronic **business card** ready to exchange with those you want to keep in contact with. Try to get a list of participants in the meeting, with their addresses. After the meeting, try to find a **few minutes to reflect alone** on what you wanted to achieve at that meeting, what actually happened, and what you can learn from this to make your next meeting better than your last.

Key Points

- Use meetings as a way to extend your work networks, and actively introduce yourself to other participants
- Arrive at the meeting a little early, to speak to others and to find a suitable seat
- Read the agenda before the meeting and prepare any remarks you wish to make
- During the meeting, focus on the discussion and try not to turn to your phone or laptop
- If you wish to make a decisive comment, judge whether this is better made early or late in the discussion of that topic, for maximum impact
- Only volunteer or agree to tasks discussed at the meeting if you can do them well and if you wish to do so for a clear reason
- Use nonverbal as well as verbal behaviour to indicate support for the comments of colleagues
- Notice at the meeting examples of good or poor practice from others in how to behave at a meeting – points that you can learn from

CHAPTER 15

How to Write a Report of a Meeting

It has been said that if there is no note to record a meeting, then that meeting never took place. Although this is not always true, it is important to have some type of **written account** of meetings of any importance. This chapter offers advice on making effective meeting notes. Other relevant chapters are noted below.

The 'Five Ws'

As we mention in the chapter on taking part in video meetings, a useful starting point in deciding what to include in a meeting report are the journalist's 'five Ws': **who, what, where, when and why**.

WHO WAS AT THE MEETING?

Who attended the meeting, who sent apologies and who simply did not attend? Often it helps to know who was present to understand what was said or, more importantly, who was present when specific decisions were taken. For more formal meetings, the note can also add what other roles were played by the participants. It is usual to also include a list of participants, indicating who was the chairperson and who prepared the report.

WHAT WAS THE CONTENT OF THE MEETING?

For formal meetings there will be an agenda with items for discussion, and a simple way to **summarise what happened** at the meeting is to use the numbered agenda items for the structure of the report. It is often useful to attach the draft agenda to the report. A clear way to understand the content of each item of the agenda is to **indicate whether the item is on the agenda 'for information', 'for discussion' or** 'for decision'. It is also usual that the chairperson introduces the agenda and tells the participants what is expected to happen in relation to each of the items on the agenda. It is the chairperson's right to indicate in which order the items will be discussed, possibly starting with those of particular importance.

WHERE DID THE MEETING TAKE PLACE?

Was this an in-person, online or hybrid meeting? For meetings with a physical location, where was this? If the location is especially significant, briefly say why.

WHEN WAS THE MEETING?

A note of a meeting may lose most of its value if the **date on which the meeting took place** is not clearly stated. Especially for repeated meetings, such as those of standing committees, it can be very important that the sequence of discussions leading to decisions can be followed, especially if there is later any dispute or challenge to a far-reaching decision. For time-sensitive issues, for example, related to an embargo, the time, as well as the date, of the meeting can be stated.

WHY DID THE MEETING TAKE PLACE?

This is perhaps the most important element in the report of a meeting. **What was the purpose of the meeting**? Was this purpose clear to all participants? Does the meeting report provide enough information for the reader to know if the meeting succeeded in achieving its aims?

Format of the Report

For most purposes, reports of meetings are most useful if they are brief and only contain vital information. The **headings can directly reflect the items on the agenda** for that meeting. This correspondence with the agenda can also extend to making clear in the report whether each item was included in the meeting for information, discussion or decision. **If decisions were made, these need to be noted** very clearly, and it may be necessary to note whether a decision was made unanimously or by consensus (where a dissenting minority of people at the meeting nevertheless decided not to block the view of the majority). In our view it is usually not necessary in a meeting report to note who said what. It is the comments themselves that are materially important. An exception may be where a meeting splits evenly on an important decision and the chair casts a deciding vote, and this process should be noted on a named person basis.

Noting Action Points

The most important aspect of the note of a meeting is to **record decisions and what actions will be taken**. For each action point, we suggest that the meeting note makes clear: (1) who will be responsible for undertaking the action; (2) by when will it be completed or if there will be an update to the meeting; (3) if some type of support is needed for the action to take place, what resources will be allocated and by whom the action will be completed; and (4) the line of accountability, namely how, to whom and when the responsible person or group will report back on progress with this action. An example of the minutes of a formal meeting is shown below.

Minutes of the ABC Board Meeting of (Date)

Time	Item
15.00	1. **Welcome**
15.05	2. **Introduction**
	Note of any conflicts of interest
	1. Overview of today's agenda
	2. Approval of the draft minutes of the last meeting
	3. List of actions from previous meeting that are not yet completed
15.10	3. **Quarter 1 Chief Executive Officer (CEO) update**
	• ACTION 1
	• Questions 1
	• Responses 1
	• ACTION 2
	• Questions 2
	• Responses 2
	• CEO SUMMARY
15.25	4. **Fundraising**
	Fundraising Officer presented their annual report on fund raising outcomes
	Successes and challenges identified – performance in line with expectations
	Funding raising plan for the next 3 years presented
	ACTION 1. Fund raising plan approved.
	ACTION 2. Investment in special reserve fund approved.
	ACTION 3. Due diligence proposal for funding prospect approved.
15.50	5. **Programme update**
	• The Chief Operating Officer (COO) gave the annual report on the scope of work and the achievements in the last financial year
	• The Board noted the quality and quantity of work undertaken, congratulated the COO and the whole team on these achievements and approved the report
15.55	6. **Thanks and close**
Papers	**Papers**
	1. List of appendices circulated for the meeting
	2. List of working papers made available to members of the Board on request

Most of the reports of meetings reflect what was presented and what decisions were taken. The meetings are prepared in draft and the draft is usually shown to the participants before it is finalised so that they can make their comments about the text. The meeting report thus records what happened and what the decisions were.

On some occasions, the reports of meetings are written by participants expressing their perception of the meeting and its decisions. Such reports are **expressing the opinion** of the writers who do not ask the participants to agree with what they have written. Such reports can be about the first meeting of a sports team, a student group, a book club or a meeting to plan a retirement event. They might include notes on any humorous moments that took place and surprising parts of the discussion or notable failures of the logistical aspects. On occasion, the formal report might be accompanied by a note or letter written to inform people who could not attend the meeting about what happened, describing the mood of the meeting, whether the participants emerged from the meeting energised (or exhausted), and what the meaning of the discussion was or the decisions were, perhaps putting these issues in a wider context.

The Implications of the Meeting

At the end of the meeting, it is usually necessary for the group to decide **if another meeting is required**. For a regular meeting, participants will benefit if they have plenty of advance notice of the time, date and place of the next meeting, usually noted in the minutes of the previous meeting, sent out just after the meeting took place. The chair of the meeting will need to balance the advantage of having a regular meeting to allow the participation of group members in the ongoing business of the team or organisations, against the time taken or even wasted by having meetings without clear aims or without enough business on any particular day. The chair can win friends by occasionally cancelling meetings, preferably well in advance.

Key Points

- In the report of the meeting, include the name of the meeting, when and where it took place, who was present and what the content of the meeting was
- Brevity: make the report as short as possible to cover the essentials
- Clarity: avoid ambiguity
- Emphasise the most important issues discussed/decided
- Implications: what will/should follow the meeting – what is next?
- How can the reader obtain more information?

Practical Exercise: The 14th Balkan Games

TASK

The teacher asks all the students in the study group to read the report below. A small number of students (e.g., three to four) are also invited to each say a sentence or two, in less than 1 minute, to the group, conveying the most important points in the report. The students are given a day to prepare their report but asked not to discuss it with anyone before their presentation. Then each of the selected students makes their presentation. After the presentations have been made, the students making the presentations are each invited to comment on their own presentations. Then all students are invited to comment on any of the presentations. Finally, the teachers offer comments about how to summarise information or discover the most cogent facts in a text.

THE 14TH BALKAN GAMES

On the 15th of January 2018 at 12:30 p.m., representatives of all the Balkan countries met to discuss the organisation of the 14th Balkan Games, which was on this occasion to include judo and tightrope walking. The delegation from Greece did not agree to these additions, and it was thus not possible to hold the games because unanimity of the participating countries was necessary to do so.

The representatives of Serbia, Croatia, Bosnia and Albania were dressed in their national costumes. The representative of other countries wore their ordinary clothes. Each of the representatives had with them a team of five highly successful athletes who were brought along to organise the events in their specialities. In all, there were 60 people in attendance, in addition to four officials from a site in Austria. The delegates were seated at a table, so that they could agree on the details of the championship.

The hosts had been careful about the numbers of people attending because they did not want to find themselves at the meeting with not enough chairs. This had happened on a previous occasion and it took quite some time to acquire more chairs. The representatives had arrived the night before the meeting and were lodged in the Hotel Bristol, which is close to the airport. They were then transported to a mountain resort and told they would be meeting at the best hotel there. They had dinner together in the hotel restaurant and, during the dinner, the delegate of Greece said that he had received a letter from his government informing him that they no longer objected to the introduction of the new disciplines, which meant that there was no obstacle to the holding of the next games. During the dinner, it was announced that the weather was deteriorating and that it was likely that heavy snowfall would block the airport. It was therefore announced that transportation to the airport would be organised for the next morning, using three cars that were reserved by the Austrian delegation.

The next morning, the representatives had breakfast, which was paid for by the organisers. They then left with the athletes, who accompanied them to the airport.

The owner of hotel in which the representatives of the countries and their teams resided was upset because some of the delegations had not paid their bills. He therefore asked to see the chairperson of the organising committee, to ask him to pay the outstanding bills. The chairperson asked the owner to write to the countries in question to obtain the payment. The owner of the hotel was not happy about this but said that he would write to the countries to get payment for the bills. The total sum in question was 350 euros, mainly referring to minibar costs in the guest rooms. The minibars were not controlled regularly and so the sums in questions were not entered in the guests' bills in time.

CHAPTER 16

How to Lead a Small Working Group or Collaboration

We have taken part in, or led, many small working groups and consortia, for example, research partnerships, and this chapter distils our views about good practice in leading small collaborative working groups. Such small groups can be effective for many purposes. For example, this might be a group to carry out an administrative task within an organisation; that forms a clinical team; to carry out a research project; of members of a not-for-profit organisation to exert pressure on a government; or with a shared experience, such as people with lived experience of a mental health condition or a group of carers. In all of these types of groups it is important to participate and behave constructively, and to build good relationships with others in the group. Not all of the issues discussed in this chapter apply equally to all of these categories of groups, so we suggest you consider our comments flexibly. Related chapters are shown below.

RELATED CHAPTERS

Chapter 8. How to work with people from other cultures
Chapter 11. How to chair a meeting
Chapter 20. How to present a proposal for funding
Chapter 22. How to negotiate
Chapter 25. How to work in a small group
Chapter 26. How to reduce tension in a small group or in a meeting
Chapter 30. How to learn from the failure of a project

What Is a Collaboration?

Thinking first about a small group being assembled to carry out a research project, we see a collaboration as a group of participants who have a **common purpose** and who have **complementary skills**, and between whom **all the necessary types of expertise** are included in the group.

Why Form a Collaboration?

There are several reasons why you may wish to lead a collaboration. This may be because a **project cannot be done in any other way**, for example, a comparative international study. Or it may be difficult or impossible to **recruit a sufficiently large sample size** of participants from one study site alone. A further strong reason to establish such a consortium is because you need to **include particular specialists** in the group, for example, statisticians, health economists, social scientists or service user participation experts. If these forms of specialist knowledge are scarce, these experts may need to be identified from different research centres either nationally or internationally. A more practical reason for an international consortium is to **allow access to research funds** that are restricted to nationals of particular countries. Thinking in the longer term, some research groups will purposively include in the collaboration more experienced individuals who, through teaching, mentoring or examples, can teach more junior colleagues about research management and leadership skills.

One model to bear in mind is called the **'best team' approach**, in which the people you invite to join a consortium are known to be among the very best in their field, regardless of where they work. We prefer a modified version of this approach. If you are leading a proposal to gain funding for research, a critical period is that at which you decide who to invite to join the core research group.

We suggest you keep three criteria in mind: (1) specialists who have a **high level of expertise** in their field; (2) people who you can **trust to deliver** on their undertakings to work hard for the project; and (3) people who are known to be **collaborative** and not self-centred or narcissistic. In our experience, working groups work well when each member fulfils all of these three criteria. If you are considering inviting a person to join your team whom you have not directly worked with before, be cautious and carry out **'due diligence'**, which means asking third parties about their experience of working with the person under consideration. Unfortunately, when we have not followed our own advice, we have occasionally had the experience of a single determined and inflexible individual damaging or even destroying an otherwise highly effective working group.

It is common for staff leading applied research projects to want project results to have a beneficial impact, for example, in the fields of health or social care. For example, at the end of a project, research leaders may communicate the research results to policy makers, guideline developers, clinical practitioners or patient groups. All too often the researchers feel disappointed in the response they get, if they receive any response. Our experience leads us to conclude that if you want any particular group, for example, policy makers, to pay attention to the results of a specific project, it is most helpful to **invite the target policy makers to join** a project in some capacity at the very start of the project. This may be as members of an advisory group, or to test their information needs in a theory of change workshop, or to undertake individual interviews at an early project stage to gain a more detailed understanding of the wider policy context, new policies that are under development, and the informational needs of the specific policy makers you wish to influence. If this information is gained at an early stage of the project, the project plan may need to be modified to increase the likelihood that the final results will be aligned with health or social care policy at that later time, and this increases the chance the research results will be seen as relevant and taken seriously.

Control or Delegation?

As a team leader, or perhaps as someone learning the skills of team leadership with support and mentorship, as you design a new project you will pay attention to the aim of the work, but also to how you want the project to run, namely the structure of the project. In the **traditional hierarchical management structure**, the project director told intermediaries what to do and the latter told the junior staff what to do. This structure can achieve the aims of a project, but it does not encourage staff at the different hierarchical levels to learn or to develop their own leadership skills.

An alternative approach is called the **matrix structure**. Table 16.1 shows the overall structure of such a matrix. This is an example of a multisite project, which in this example has five **study sites**. Each site (shown in the rows of the table) has a named person to be responsible for the research activities that need to take place at that site. The project work is separated in a series of separate blocks of work called 'work packages' (WPs). Each WP is a coherent part of the research project, and all WPs need to be undertaken well for the project to succeed. Each WP has a clearly named person responsible for ensuring that this part of the project is completed and is done well. The first work package is for overall project coordination.

Staff in WP1 need to explain to each of the site leads what is expected of them, and when and with what resources. At the same time, WP1 needs to explain to WP leads what they need to do, and with whom and when. In this matrix model, each site and each WP receives a devolved budget, with which they need to achieve specific 'deliverables' to set timescales. The project coordinators will keep up a regular check to see if each set of deliverables is being completed well and to the agreed time plan. If not, then the project coordinators are to identify any variations from the project plan very early and move quickly to support the group to recover sufficient progress.

Such a matrix structure for leading and coordinating groups working on a research project can succeed extremely well through this **type of delegation**, and it gives in this case at least 10 people the opportunity to use or gain research leadership skills. The matrix structure also allows the project subgroups to be held accountable to the senior members of the project team through regular project updates. It can also be an advantage to have two named people to lead each site or each WP, both to give the option for a more junior person to learn such skills through practical experience, and also to build in some reserve resilience if, for example, a lead person needs to leave the group midway through the project. We have used this approach for global mental health projects called Emerald and Indigo in recent years.

What Has Experience Taught Us?

From our experience in leading research working groups, we feel we have learned, sometimes through mistakes or adversity, several important lessons:

When bidding for research funds, aim to offer the funder exactly what they want. This means learning what the funding body want to fund. If this is not clear from

TABLE 16.1 ■ Matrix structure for a multisite programme that has several work packages

	Work package 1 Project coordination WP lead person	Work package 2 Systematic review WP lead person	Work package 3 Formative Phase WP lead person	Work package 4 Intervention phase WP lead person	Work package 5 Knowledge transfer WP lead person
Site 1 Lead person					
Site 2 Lead person					
Site 3 Lead person					
Site 4 Lead person					
Site 5 Lead person					

the published research call for proposals, you may need to contact the funders to try to find out this information.

Follow the golden rule and treat others as you would wish to be treated. Remarkably, staff roles in working groups often change so that, for example, a junior member of staff can be rapidly promoted to a more senior role. For both ethical and pragmatic reasons, therefore, we suggest that as a research working group leader you treat all staff with utmost kindness, consideration and courtesy, not least because your current junior staff may be your own future overlord!

Provide a **high level of transparency about the budget**. We have had extensive experience in groups where the project directors have either shared budget information in detail with all lead project staff or have acted as if finances were top secret. We prefer transparency. This is to avoid suspicion of unfairness in the group and potential rivalry, but also because often, sooner or later, projects have budgetary difficulties, with a cut in the allocation to the project as a whole, some unplanned overspend, or progress to deliver results that is too slow. The project director will often need to ask for revisions to the budget and if, for example, site and work package leads have been receiving regular updates on the planned and actual expenditure for the allocated tasks, there will be a greater degree of trust to renegotiate the budgets or timetable for deliverables.

Include as much teaching and capacity building as possible. After a project has been completed, what is left behind? The project results should be completed and published as originally planned, but in fact often far fewer publications are actually completed than intended. An important aspect of the sustainability of a project are the skills acquired by staff in carrying out the research project, most importantly the 'transferrable skills' that they can use and apply in future projects and working groups. The project achievements may also strengthen the curricula vitae of early- or intermediate-career-stage staff to strengthen their opportunities for career advancement and promotion. For these reasons, we suggest in the course of running a project that you include as much capacity building as possible, including, for example, a mentorship programme.

Think of a consortium as a **long-term network of relationships**. Although the fundings for specific projects is very often time limited, during a working lifetime, human relationships are not. We encourage you to think in terms of working groups such as research consortium, not as 3–5-year projects, but as groups with the potential to enjoy collaborating and undertaking high quality work for 10 years, 20 years, or longer. Leadership roles will change over as junior staff gain experience and confidence and as senior staff may move into legacy/succession mode, but the same mutual respect personally and professionally needs to be actively maintained.

Establish and maintain a close relationship with your funder. At some stage, most funded projects experience an unexpected difficulty, which, if left unresolved, could jeopardise the whole work. This could be, for example, through a financial, political or natural disaster, crisis at a study site, or illness of a key study lead person. Whatever the nature of the problem, it is likely that the project coordinator will need to ask for some flexibility from the funder to deliver the overall aims of the project. Such discussions are much more likely to go well if there is a preexisting strong relationship with the funder. We therefore encourage project coordinators to invite funders to some project meetings, such as the initial project set-up or launch meetings; to produce regular and attractive project newsletters; and to involve funders in other active ways, both to assure them that the project is going well, and as a precaution in case core details of the project may need to be renegotiated at some stage. If a costed or no-cost extension to the duration of the project may be necessary, try to give as much advance notice of this as possible to the funder.

Understand the needs and constraints of project partners. As the leader of a working group, you will meet colleagues in your team who are underperforming for different reasons. Try to get to know each key individual in your team on a personal basis. In our experience there is no substitute to meeting in-person with colleagues for forming and maintaining close relationships. This is particularly important at the start of projects and when serious problems arise, and the latter can be much harder to resolve by remote communication than by an in-person meeting. We have noted that during the periods of lockdown and travelling restrictions that were imposed during the COVID-19 pandemic of 2020–2023, the quality of the interpersonal relationships tended to deteriorate without such in-person meetings. Once good working relationships have been established, routine communications can usually be managed well with regular phone or video meetings. These can be supplemented from time to time with short internal newsletters, especially to note achievements. Try hard to celebrate positive news within the team. We often start project meeting with an item about 'good news'.

Identify critical points of conflict early on and prevent or mitigate them. Proposals to fund projects often have a section on 'risks to the project and mitigation plans'. This is an opportunity for those leading the project proposal to look into the future, imagine potential problems, and prepare plans to reduce the impact on the project if any of these difficulties arise. Some points of conflict or tension are entirely predictable, such as arrangements for authorship of papers (see the chapters on reading and writing research papers). We have found that having a clear, written set of rules about authorship of research papers, agreed at the beginning of each project, can be enormously helpful to avoid later, and sometimes poisonous, publication disagreements. This contract can be signed by all partners, and then lead to a specific publication plan for each project, in which each developing publication is named, the members of the writing group are named, and a timescale for drafting the papers is agreed. This plan can be discussed, for example, every month or every 2 months at project team meetings.

Keep in mind the key characteristics of more effective teams. Staff at Google have investigated which characteristics seem to be most closely linked with more effective teams. Fig. 16.1 shows their findings.

- **Psychological safety** was found to be the most effective element. This allows staff to take risks, to feel comfortable with sharing vulnerability and uncertainty,

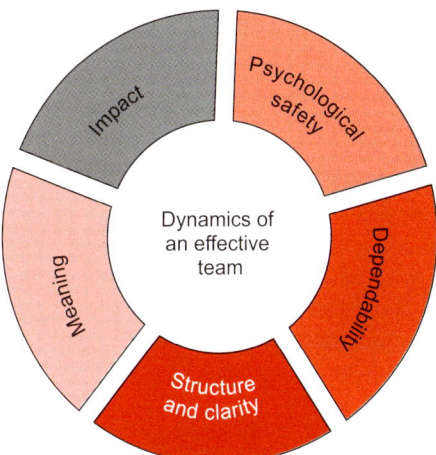

Fig. 16.1   Five key characteristic of effective teams. From: https://www.thinkwithgoogle. com/intl/en-gb/consumer-insights/consumer-trends/five-dynamics-effective-team/.

to be able to admit making mistakes and to feeling confident about offering new ideas.

- **Dependability:** In dependable teams, team members reliably complete quality work on time. This is both very simple and very important for effective team functioning.
- **Structure and clarity:** In a highly effective team there are clear roles, goals and plans that are understood by all team members. Individuals understand what is expected of the whole, what is expected of them individually, and how specific contributions will combine to achieve the whole team's goals.
- **Meaning:** Team members need to feel that the work being undertaken has a purpose that they value. As individuals are different, so the meaning the work has for different team members will also vary.
- **Impact:** Can team members clearly see that their project work is making a difference in some important respect? Are their individual and group efforts sufficiently recognised in achieving their intended impact?

Successful team meetings. Successful teams tend to hold successful team meetings, at least most of the time. We have noticed two specific ways in which strong teams communicate internally. First, the available time for the meeting is relatively equally shared between all those present. In other words, no one person or small group will dominate the 'air time'. Second, the content of team meetings is both transactional (about the technical details of the work to be done) and relational (team members express their emotions about the work and its impact upon them). Wise team leaders or those chairing team meetings may therefore actively support contributions from all team members, as well as legitimising the expression of technical information and the feelings of team members.

Key Points

- If you lead in forming a collaboration, we suggest you consider group members who fulfil these criteria: (1) specialists who have a high level of expertise in their field; (2) people who you can trust to deliver on their undertakings to work hard for the project; and (3) people who are known to be collaborative and not self-centred or narcissistic
- Be very cautious about inviting people to join the group if you do not know if they meet most or all of these criteria
- Decide with the consortium early on about the type of leadership to use for the work of the group, for example, a more traditional, directive approach by the leader, or one of delegated responsibility to people leading key components of the programme
- When bidding for research funds, aim to offer the funder exactly what they want
- Follow the golden rule and treat others as you would wish to be treated
- Include as much teaching and capacity building as possible
- Establish and maintain a close relationship with your funder
- Understand the needs and constraints of project partners
- Identify critical points of conflict early on and prevent or mitigate them

CHAPTER 17

How to Interview Candidates for a Job or Position

From a relatively early stage of your career you may be asked to join a panel or committee to interview candidates for a job or position. This could be, for example, because the chair of the committee wants to include people of your status in the organisation to balance the composition of the committee, or because of the skills or experience you have. Related chapters are shown below. This chapter offers you information about how to prepare for this, and how to take part in such a meeting as an interviewer.

RELATED CHAPTERS

Chapter 18. How to behave in an interview for a post
Chapter 37. How to apply for a post

Preparing for the Interview

When you are invited to take part in an interview as an interviewer, check that you **understand the nature of the invitation**. What will your role be? Will you be involved in all stages of the appointment? Will you be involved in both the shortlisting and interviewing of candidates? Note that for some posts there can be very many applicants, so that assessing all applications to decide on who should be shortlisted can be very time consuming. Will you have the same influence on the appointment decision as other committee members? Are you being invited to join the committee in a personal capacity or to represent another body such as junior practitioners in your speciality or discipline?

Then look carefully at the **details of the job or post**. Often there will be a job description and a person specification available to the candidates and the interview committee. Sometimes more details are available, for example, 'further particulars'.

Next, **plan for the day of the interview**. What is the date and what is the time? Read the application documents of all the shortlisted candidates whom you will interview, make your notes about their strengths and weaknesses, and list what you see as the main questions or issues to clarify for each person. Note any potentially important gaps in each CV that you may want to explore during the interview.

Think in advance, in case you are asked for your views about which questions you would like to ask during the interview. The chair may allocate two or three questions to you about whatever you would like to focus upon.

Prepare your papers so that you can **make brief notes** about each question for each candidate during the interview, and check to see if there is a standard scoring system set by your human resources department to rate candidates on particular domains or capabilities.

If your organisation has a particular **policy on how to conduct interviews**, read this carefully and be sure that you follow the correct way to conduct the interview. This may refer, for example, to equal opportunities arrangements designed to avoid bias or discrimination in the recruitment process, and some employers insist on asking all the candidates exactly the same questions and only these questions.

Also check in advance if there is a specific way to **record how you assess each candidate**. Often there is a marking system, either for each question or for each domain or skill being assessed, which asks you, for example, to rate for each category if the candidate exceeds, meets or fails to meet the required standard.

Arriving at the Interview

Arrive early. Informally meet all the members of the interview panel, **introduce yourself** and try to find out where they work and what they are looking for in the successful candidate. As the meeting starts, expect the chair of the panel to introduce everyone, to explain briefly the post that has been advertised, and to indicate what qualities the successful candidate is expected to demonstrate. The chair may also check if there are any actual or potential conflicts of interest by panel members. Usually the chair will appoint one of the panel to make notes of the meeting and of the appointment decision, but if this is not clear you may need to gently ask at the beginning of the meeting who will make notes of the most important issues and decisions.

The chair is likely to propose a **plan for how the interview will take place**. Will there be an initial presentation by each candidate? Who will ask which questions in which sequence? Usually this will be to set a series of key questions, e.g., between six and ten, with two or three questions allocated to each committee member. Clearly this will be different if you alone will interview the candidates. Will all the candidates be seen on the same day? What happens if some candidates do not attend the interview? Will the discussion about the appointment take place immediately after the interviews and will decisions be taken on the same day about who to offer the post to?

It may be important to check in advance of the interviews, for internal candidates, if any **prior knowledge** or experience by panel members can be brought into the discussion. Some organisations do not allow this, to try to be fair to external candidates. Find out before the interviews start about how long has been allocated for each interview.

During the Interview

It is good practice for the chair to **greet each candidate** as they enter the room, to introduce each member of the committee, and perhaps to offer a glass of water. Keep in mind that this interview may be a very important event for the candidate, with a lot at stake in terms of their career or employment, and they may be very nervous. Try to put candidates at their ease early in the meeting. Often it is helpful to allow the candidate to relax a little by asking a relatively easy question to start with such as 'Please tell us why you have applied for this position'.

Some interviews invite candidates to make an **initial brief statement or presentation** about their application, for example, up to 5 minutes, perhaps with slides, on their background, their proposal, their key strengths or their track record. If this is the case, keep to time.

During the interview, notice how other members of the panel ask their questions and if they are continuously courteous and kind to the applicants, whether or not they are impressing you during the interview. See if the chair allows follow-up or **supplementary questions** from panel members if they want greater detail on any topic or if they want to press a very good candidate.

Note whether the chair allows discussion by the panel after each candidate, as sometimes no discussion is allowed until after all the candidates have been seen.

During each interview, decide for yourself (1) if the candidate is **appointable or not** and why, and (2), if you think the person is appointable, whether this application is moderately good, strong or very strong, and why. Make brief notes to support your views on each issue to be used in the later discussion.

During each interview consider (and make notes on) **what** each candidate says in answer to each question, **how** the candidate expresses themselves (with passion or detachment), any issues that they seem to want to avoid or **downplay**, and if there are any **inconsistencies** between what they say and what is on their CV or application form.

Has the candidate dressed appropriately for a formal occasion? Does the candidate give the impression that they have prepared thoroughly for the interview – for both this particular post and in relation to this organisation? Are their answers to interview questions specifically tailored to this particular job? Does the candidate give the impression that they **really do want this job** without any hesitation or ambivalence? Does the candidate seem to be **genuine and sincere** throughout the meeting? If the **candidate asks any questions** of the panel, are these thoughtful and do they strengthen a positive impression of the person?

After the Interview

Now comes the decision point. You need to know if you are a full 'voting member' of the committee; if not, you may be there as an observer or a nonvoting member, so be sure of your status. The chair may ask for initial **brief comments from all panel members** about the relative strengths and weaknesses of the candidates who have been interviewed. Be prepared for this first round of discussion. At this stage, do not go into too much detail about your views but do say if you think that any candidates are **not appointable**.

The chair will usually try to get **agreement or consensus** among the panel members of who is not seen to be appointable, and who is therefore excluded from further consideration. For the candidates remaining for discussion, there will usually be a round of more detailed discussions. Be vigilant in case you feel that the views of any panel member may be unfairly biased for or against particular candidates, and if you disagree with any statement, gently ask the person to give specific reasons for the points they express. If you are a full member of the committee, do be confident in challenging, very politely, any point of view with which you disagree, especially if you can refer to your notes and give strong supporting arguments for your point of view.

Try to avoid making a definitive statement about your **preference on who to appoint** too early. Assess the feelings of the committee members to see if consensus is emerging. When a preferred candidate is selected, check that the chair also identifies if there is an appointable **reserve candidate**, in case the first-choice person does not accept the job offer.

During the discussion, see if you can **learn from other committee members** about how they assess the different aspects of the candidate's strengths and weaknesses and whether you agree with their analyses or not. Be sure that it is clear **who will contact the preferred candidate** and provide feedback to the other panel members on whether the preferred candidate accepts the position or not.

Also **clarify what the job offer entails** – is this for full time or part time work? When is the start date? What is the salary? How much is the person expected to physically be in the office? Are there any other factors that need to be declared or discussed, such as disability or known periods of future absence from work, and is negotiation on these issues possible? Are there **particular conditions** that the candidate needs to meet or demonstrate before the appointment can be confirmed?

If the committee comes to the view that **none of the candidates is appointable**, what is the plan? The chair needs to agree who will inform the candidates of the outcome of the interviews and what the next step is. Will the post be advertised again and in the same way? Or will it be modified to try and attract stronger candidates? If a formal marking system was used, the score sheets of each committee member need to be collected, either by an administrator or by the chair.

It is good practice, in **closing the meeting**, for the chair to thank the committee members for their contributions to the meeting and to show that they value the time of the panel members. Also, the chair should inform the committee members later **if the preferred candidate has accepted the post**, while adding a further written note thanking the panel for their contributions. As you leave the meeting, perhaps **reflect on what you have learned** that can help you the next time that you are on an interview committee, and also the next time you apply for a post and are interviewed yourself.

Key Points

- If you are invited to join an interview panel, read the invitation carefully to understand what you are being invited to do
- Before the interview day, read all the applications and make brief notes about the strengths and weaknesses of each candidate and what you would like to ask each person
- Before the interview starts, find out if that company or organisation has a particular policy on how interviews should be conducted and how the views of the interview panel are recorded
- On arriving at the interview, meet other panel members and check that the chair is clear about who will do what during the interviews
- For each candidate, decide if you think they are appointable, and for those who are, rank them in order of strength of application and interview
- Be prepared to give your views clearly and to listen carefully to the views of others during the discussion after the interview. Be sure to check that the contingency is discussed of what will be done if the preferred candidate does not accept the post
- Watch carefully what other members of the interview panel do and see what you can learn from them

CHAPTER 18

How to Behave in an Interview for a Post

At particular stages of your career you will probably apply for work posts or for particular opportunities, such as clinical or research fellowships or research positions, where the first stage consists of submitting an application form or curriculum vitae (see Chapter 32). You may then be selected to attend an interview as a part of the selection process. This chapter offers information about preparing for an interview, how to behave during the interview, and what to do after the interview. Related chapters are shown below.

What Is an Interview?

The meaning of interview has changed over recent centuries. From the early 16th century, the terms meant a **face-to-face meeting**, from the French word *entrevue* meaning 'to see each other, visit each other briefly, have a glimpse of'. Its modern meaning usually refers to a **personal meeting to discuss employment**.

Preparation for the Interview

The phrase '**By failing to prepare, you are preparing to fail**' is usually attributed to Benjamin Franklin, and this contains an important truth. In our view, most of what you can do for an interview takes place before the actual meeting, in the preparation phase. **Very careful and detailed preparation** will be very likely to improve your performance on the day. We suggest the following types of preparation.

Check and double **check** the date and time of the interview, and exact venue where the interview will take place. If the place is unfamiliar to you, then consider visiting it before the interview so you know exactly where to go. It is often the case that finding a large clinic or hospital or university is unproblematic, but finding the correct building, floor or room is not straightforward.

If you can, find out beforehand who is on the interview panel. You may need to contact the secretariat of the organisation holding the interview to get this information. Do homework to find out about the **members of the interview panel**. What are their current and recent positions? What types of expertise do they have? Do any of your colleagues or friends know these people and what can they tell you about them? Try to find a few positive aspects of their work and mention these at the interview without being excessively sycophantic.

Speak to people who have been interviewed before. If possible, find out the types of questions that will be asked or what areas will be asked about. Find out how long the interview is expected to last. **Arrive early** and have plenty of time, to minimise any avoidable anxiety on the day. Sit down at least several days before the interview and write down the questions you expect that you will be asked at the interview. Then write down key points you will want to make for each question. Ask friends and colleagues for the questions that they expect you will be asked. Also prepare answers to those questions in bullet point form.

If you may be anxious during the interview and forget some of your preprepared answers, **write down your notes on index cards, note paper, or on your phone or tablet**, and refer to this during the interview. Plan what clothes you will wear and make sure that they will be clean and presentable on the day, along with recent attention to your hairstyle. Plan to **dress rather more formally** than usual – it is better to be 'overdressed' than 'underdressed'. The interviewer will note that you have seen the interview as important and that you are keen to be selected. If you need to travel long-distance to the interview, try to **travel on the day before** the interview to have some reserve time. Assume you will have travel delays.

Arrange with family, friends or colleagues to **do live mock interviews**. Start these as far ahead of the real interview as possible so you have time to revise your preparation, and then have more mock interviews. You tell them which questions to ask, and you can suggest that they press you quite hard during these preparatory sessions. Try to make these 'dry run' interviews even harder than you expect the real interview to be.

Be sure to **ask for frank feedback** after these mock interviews and take comments seriously. You may need to revise what you plan to say to a minor or a major degree, depending on the feedback you receive. If possible, **audio- or video-record these mock interviews** and then listen to or watch yourself, making notes about what you can improve. Although you will probably have sent a CV, letter of motivation, and/or application form for the post already, be aware that the purpose of that stage was simply to get you an interview.

The interview stage is mostly unrelated to the application/CV stage and requires different skills.

As you prepare what you plan to say, think about **how your application will stand out** from those of other applicants – in business jargon, what are your unique selling points'? What do you want the interview panel to remember from your interview and how will you plan to communicate your key points to have this impact?

Read the job description and person specification for the post several times and from these documents make a list of characteristics that the panel will enquire about. **Make a table** and for every point mentioned write down your experience or qualification that shows that you satisfy or exceed each criterion – while being wholly truthful about your accomplishments.

At the Interview

Remember basic elements of **good interpersonal skills**: address panel members formally and by name, and maintain eye contact with the members of the panel all the time. Remain calm and courteous throughout the whole interview, even if you think you are being treated harshly – do not argue with any panel member. Sit up straight in your chair and lean slightly forward with your weight on the balls of your feet under your chair, as if you were about to stand up. If you need to make an initial presentation to summarise your application, for example, if you are using **PowerPoint slides, practice your presentation carefully in advance**, making sure that you **do not exceed the allocated time**, and tend to simplify the number of slides and the slide content (see Chapter 2).

For a presentation, keep in mind the specific people on the interview panel before deciding what level of detail to use in your initial talk. If you are asked a question that you do not fully understand, gently ask the panel member to rephrase or paraphrase the question so that you are sure you understand it. If you are asked a rather general or abstract question, try to give a short general answer and then immediately strengthen your answer by **giving specific examples** of your experience that show that you meet this criterion. Do **refer to your actual experiences**, for example, in clinical or research settings, especially those that are recent.

You may not know early in the interview if the panel prefer you to give short or long answers, so tend to give shorter answers, and then, if you do have more relevant detail to offer, ask 'Would you like me to go into more detail on this topic?'. Only give relevant information in each answer – do not move your answer away from the question. **Do not bluff**. If you do not know the answer to a question, say so and, even better, say that you will look into this after the interview and send a written answer on this point to the interview panel if they wish.

If you are applying for a research-related post, show a strong clinical or scientific curiosity about the work of the position being advertised. Include references (this means the name of the person cited and year of the reference) to what you have read recently, or to experts you have heard recently on the specific work topics or have met recently. Tend to be very polite and thank each panel member for each question. Do not, however, start some of your answers by saying 'This is an excellent question', because it immediately suggests that other prior questions were in your opinion not very good questions. Keep in mind the main strengths you have that you want the panel to understand and remember, and be sure to mention them at least once during the interview. In your examples of your experience, also convey to the panel, directly or indirectly, that **you work well in teams** and that you enjoy collaboration.

Avoid overly flamboyant hand or body gestures or sitting too rigidly and still. Keep hand and arm gestures moderate and symmetrical. Keep a friendly expression and, if you can, smile appropriately and quite often, without overdoing this. Do not use jokes at any point of the interview, nor satire or irony. In your answers do refer to detailed sections of your CV, application or letter of motivation, when this is relevant. **Show enthusiasm** for the post you are applying for and show passion for the work to be undertaken in the new post. If your post needs you to have skills at a level that you do not yet possess, make this clear in what you say and mention your plan for how you want to acquire these skills – show that you are committed to 'lifelong learning'.

Accentuate the positive at all times. Do not criticise any current or former colleagues. If asked about any gaps in your CV, give a brief and honest statement, preferably one that you have previously prepared. If you are asked an especially difficult or complex question, you may wish to repeat or paraphrase the question to give yourself a moment or two to compose your reply. If a panel member makes a valid criticism of your application, accept this graciously.

At the end of the interview, it is common for the committee chair to ask if there is anything else you would like to say or if you have any questions. Time is usually very short, so it is better not to have any questions, for example, you can say that the job description is very clear. Do not ask when you will receive the result of the interview. This tends to annoy panel members as they do not know yet if they will quickly agree on the interview result or not. **Express your thanks** to the panel for the interview. For video interviews, special preparation is needed, so make careful preparations bearing in mind the element of good practice for video meetings, set out in Chapter 19.

Please see Table 18.1 for frequently asked questions during an interview.

TABLE 18.1 ■ **Frequently asked questions during an interview**

- Why have you applied for this post?
- What are your qualifications for this post?
- What sets you apart from other applicants for this position?
- What relevant experience do you have that makes you a strong candidate for this post?
- Give us an example of your specialist knowledge or a recent complex challenge in your work setting and describe how you responded.
- What about this particular post is especially attractive or interesting to you?
- Would you need training to support you to succeed in this post?
- What are your limitations or weaknesses in relation to this particular post?
- What are your career plans and intentions?

After the Interview

If at all possible, **seek feedback** from the panel about your performance at the interview, whether or not you were successful. In particular, say that you would be grateful to receive written feedback so that you can reflect on this after your elation or disappointment at the interview result has subsided, so that you can learn to do even better at future interviews.

Key Points

- Prepare very thoroughly for each interview you attend
- Prepare in detail for the specific post or opportunity you are applying for and read and reread the relevant documents
- Try to find out who will interview you and get background information on them
- Prepare index cards or equivalent with probably questions and the outline of your preprepared answers
- Know exactly where and when your interview is and arrive early
- Practice mock interviews several times with friends, family and colleagues
- Dress formally
- During the interview remain calm and courteous – do not use humour
- If you do not understand a question, ask for it to be paraphrased
- If you do not know the answer to a question, say so honestly
- Try to find opportunities to mention and emphasise your particular strengths
- Tend not to ask questions at the end of the interview, even if you are invited to do so

Practical Exercise

Three members of the group are invited to prepare for an interview for a special fellowship, lasting for year, at a centre of excellence at a particular prestigious university or hospital. Each fellowship can be to learn a new clinical or research skill. In front of the group, a teacher conducts a one-to-one interview in turn with the three group members. The teacher is likely to ask each applicant what they propose to do and why, and when they propose to do it. Questions may also address if each candidate has been in touch with the centre of excellence and has an agreement in principle to have a visiting attachment. The interview can close with questions about how the fellowship would assist the career development of each candidate and what the benefits would be to other people. The second and third interviewees should stay in a separate nearby room while the earlier interviews take place. After the third interview, the interviewees join the main group. Except for the interviewees, the group is then asked to write down their single preference for the winning candidate. The group is asked for their views on the three interview performances. The interviewer is then asked for their first preference for the fellowship and why. The results of the group votes for the fellowship are then announced. The candidates are then invited to comment on their own experience of the interview and their performance. There is then a period of general discussion by the whole group on the potentially differing priorities for the fellowship and the criteria used in making these decisions. The session finishes with the teachers making a summary to synthesise key learning points.

CHAPTER 19

How to Take Part in a Video Meeting

Video meetings were less common for professional purposes until the COVID-19 pandemic began in 2020. Restricted travel and lockdown arrangements saw a huge increase in the use of video and online ways to communicate, for example, with colleagues, clients or patients. This chapter offers information on good practice in taking part in video meetings, but the points discussed in the chapter need to be applied flexibly because meetings will vary, for example, in relation to the country in which they take place, if they are one-off or a repeated series of meetings, if they are consultations, or if they are congress style meetings such as symposia, workshops or round tables. Related chapters are shown below.

RELATED CHAPTERS

Preparing for a Video Meeting

You will need the same information as you prepare for a meeting as that needed by a journalist writing a factual article – often called the 'five Ws'.

- **Who** is the host, and who are the presenters and participants? Find out who is organising the meeting, who is making a presentation and who is likely to attend the meeting, and find out more about their backgrounds. Anticipate their contributions on the basis of their track record of work or achievements.
- **What** is the content of the meeting? Get background papers on the meeting agenda or any advance notices or flyers, to know as much as possible before the meeting starts.
- **Where** will the meeting take place? On which video platform will the meeting take place? Are you familiar with this, for example, in using screen share in this particular programme? Do you need to practice this? If you have not used the

programme for a while, will it need some time before starting to update itself and have you allowed time for this, especially if you have an important role at the meeting?
- **When** will the meeting be held: at what time, in what time zone, on what date, and for what duration? Check the start and finish time for your time zone and for other participants if you are the meeting organiser or host. Be cautious in the spring and autumn when clock changes can alter the relative times between time zones. If you are the host, will the video meeting stop automatically at the end time for the meeting or will it allow you continue to meet if the meeting runs over time?
- **Why**: what is the purpose of meeting? Is there a clear aim of the meeting on behalf of the organiser? If not, for potentially important meetings, do you want to contact the host in advance to ask for details of the aim of the meeting? Do different participants in the meeting have different aims in terms of what they want to achieve?

Preparation if You Are Hosting the Meeting

As for any meeting, tell participants well in advance, and at least a week in advance for formal meetings, about the **time and location of the meeting**, with clear instructions for which internet weblinks to use to join the meeting. If the video platform is not one that people are familiar with, ask participants to download the programme or app and to practise using it. Be clear about the meeting times in all relevant world time zones. Be cautious about posting weblinks to the meeting on public platforms or social media, to reduce the risk of malicious attacks on your meeting. Give **clear instructions to speakers about who is speaking**, in what order the presentations will take place and how long each speaker has to speak. Often it will be helpful to **start the meeting about 15 minutes early** so that speakers can join before the main meeting starts to check the practical arrangements such as screen share. Ask permission of the speakers if the meeting can be recorded and tell them why you want to record it. For larger meetings you may want to use some of the advanced video meeting options, such as having a separate speakers'room', so that they can 'move' between this and the main meeting. Check for each speaker if these options are clear and work well.

For a larger meeting as host you may well want to **appoint one or two meeting moderators** to help you. For example, they can keep an eye on the chats or on the question and answer section, to feed key points to you to bring into a discussion. Test before the meeting how you will communicate in this way, for example, using direct chats or text messages.

Before the meeting starts, check that you have enough information to correctly introduce the speakers and check with each speaker **how to pronounce their name** and if the information you have is correct and up to date. Rehearse in advance your greeting to all participants when the meeting starts, what you will say to open the meeting, what you will say to introduce the purpose and the structure of the meeting, and how you will introduce the speakers.

Unless you are sure that meeting participants will follow a reasonable protocol, **spell out the etiquette for the meeting**, for example, muting microphones when not speaking, whether you prefer participants to have their video cameras on or off during the meeting or when speaking, and whether to ask people to 'raise a hand' when wanting to speak or if you will allow spontaneous comments from participants. Where wi-fi bandwidth is poor or variable for some participants, communication may be clearer by using sound only and switching off all cameras. If a presenter or a speaker loses connection, try to bring them into the meeting again later when they reconnect. Try hard to keep to the timetable for the meeting and in particular stop speakers exceeding their time allocations.

For most meetings it can be helpful to **expect that everyone at the meeting may be able to make a helpful contribution** if allowed or encouraged to do so. Consider pausing at several points during the meeting for comments or questions, and you may wish to ask for comments particularly from people who have not already spoken. As the host or chair of a meeting, follow the usual guidelines for meetings, whether in-person or online, in being courteous throughout, being clear with participants which item on the agenda is being discussed, offering some time for discussion for most issues, and summarising each discussion and clarifying any actions points before moving on to the next agenda item (see Chapter 11).

Preparation if You Are Presenting at the Meeting

If you are invited to a meeting, is it clear **who the organiser or host** is? If you want to make a presentation, has the host given you **permission to use the 'share screen' function**, preferably in advance rather than during the meeting? For important meetings, join early to test sharing your screen and showing presentation in full screen mode, to ensure that this works well and quickly when you go live. Before the meeting, check if you have a direct way to contact the host, in case there is any problem in connecting to the video meeting.

Even if you are not presenting or hosting the meeting, it can be a good idea to **join 5 or 10 minutes early** to greet other participants and to have informal discussions. One of the major disadvantages of video meetings is that the informal time to gossip or catch up with colleagues before or after in-person meetings is usually lost. Try to create other ways for informal, as well as formal, communication via video. Before you join the meeting, check that the screen will display your name during the video conference.

If you are going to make a presentation at the meeting, **prepare carefully**, for example, by shutting down any other open programmes on your computer that might cause embarrassment if you shared the wrong screen with your colleagues. Often it can help to start the meeting if participants introduce themselves to others using the chat function as they join the meeting, sending this to all participants. If you need to check some aspect of the meeting arrangements, you can use the chat option to send a direct message only to the host.

Before starting your presentation, check with the hosts if they will show your slides or documents or if you will. If the hosts **control the slides**, test that this works before the meeting starts and that they have the correct version of the slides you want to show. Test saying 'next slide' and that one of the hosts advances the slides correctly. At the end of each presentation it is helpful to end the screen share promptly. Remember to include a clear first slide with your own details and the title/aim of your presentation, and to include your name and contact details on your last slide, which you can show for long enough for people to make a note if they want to contact you.

Make careful preparations that your **audio and visual settings** work well, especially if you are a presenter. Using a headset with an attached microphone will often give the best quality sound, whereas attached speaker phones or inbuilt computer microphone and loudspeakers give poorer quality sound and are more prone to sound feedback. Inbuilt computer video cameras can work well but external video cameras often provide better picture quality. These are often pre-set to expect low light intensity, so the picture will be clearer and sharper if you can add direct natural light coming to your face from the front or from inexpensive lights you can set up on your desktop. Avoid having bright light directly overhead, which can accentuate the contours of your face in an unflattering way or bright light behind you, which can cause a silhouette effect so that your face is in shadow to viewers.

Prepare the **accessories** you need in advance: a glass of water if you may be nervous or anxious, and a notepad to take down details of key issues or action points from the meeting. If there is a noisy lawn mower in the neighbourhood, shut your windows in advance. If possible, make arrangements to reduce pet sounds or pets visible to meeting participants, unless you deliberately want to create this effect. You may wish to share aspects of your private life with everyone online, and small, furry creatures are often very effective in breaking the ice in newly forming groups! See Fig. 19.1.

During the Meeting

Check what **picture others will have of you** during the meeting. Be sure that your clothes that others can see are appropriate for the meeting. If you do show a picture of your surroundings, consider if you want all the meeting participants to see where you are, especially if you join the meeting from home. If your camera has a zoom function, check that this does not show a picture of your face that is too large or too small. Try to avoid having your video camera too low so that your face shows a large chin against a background of your ceiling. It is usually better to arrange for your camera to be at eye level.

Be careful in what you say. Some ways of expressing yourself, such as irony or sarcasm, may work in-person if others can see the disjunction between your verbal and nonverbal behaviour, but this may be more difficult to interpret on camera. In general, avoid humour for larger meetings unless you understand the group and the context well, and even then tend to use only self-deprecating humour. A joke that is misunderstood or goes wrong can cause offence.

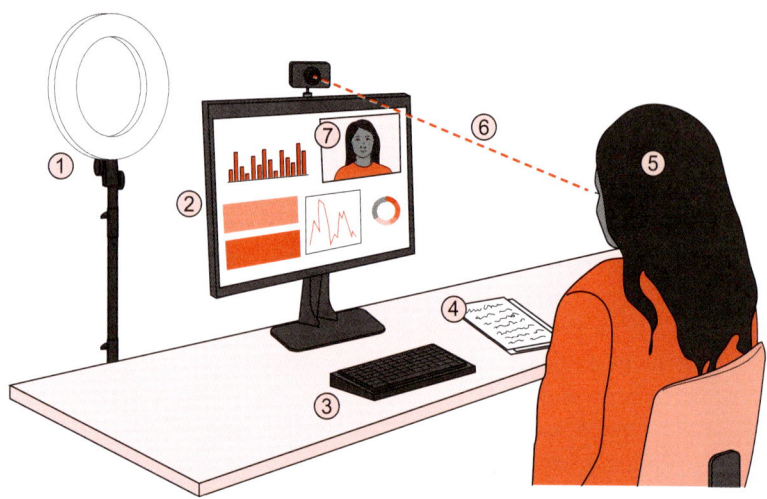

Fig. 19.1 Key points to consider when preparing for a video meeting. *(1) Shows a light near the screen monitor to illuminate the video participant's face from the front; (2) screen/monitor (3) keyboard (4) notes/papers for the participants (5) participant (6) line of sight so the participant can look at the camera (on top of the screen) and so seem to look directly at other video meeting participants (7) picture of this participant on his/he screen that other participants will see – to check that it is centred and not too close up or distant.*

Eye contact is a problem during video meetings. At in-person meetings we tend to use eye contact as one way to judge another person, and people often have views about what is too much or too little eye contact. In video meetings, eye contact is indirect and has a somewhat artificial feeling. This is especially the case if some participants at a meeting use two computer screens and seem to look at other participants relatively rarely. The best proxy for eye contact is to look directly as the camera most of the time, especially when speaking or when being spoken to directly. Poor quality cameras or low light conditions may mean that you will need to exaggerate nonverbal gestures such as nodding or smiling to some extent, but without grossly overexaggerating.

Familiarise yourself with the options for **screen gestures** such as raise hand, applause or various emotional icons. Remember to lower your 'hand' after making your comment. Check early in the meeting if there is any delay or lag in what people say, or in any of the video programme functions such a muting/unmuting, and allow for this. If people repeatedly interrupt or speak over each other for these reasons, ask for a pause after each comment before the next contribution. Many studies show that participants tend to rate video meetings as more stressful than in-person meetings, so tend to make video meetings relatively short and do what you can to maintain a positive emotional tone. If there are points of conflict, these may need to be dealt with separately, for example, in a subsequent smaller video meeting or in-person, to aim for a resolution.

After the Meeting

Assume that any **microphone is live** unless you are sure that it is muted. Do not make a controversial comment, for example, about other participants at the meeting, which they may be able to hear, even if the formal meeting has finished. If you have recorded the meeting, make use of this recording promptly, for example, to write minutes of the meeting or to make the video available to agreed others. Consider if you want to have a separate subgroup meeting immediately after the main meeting, or to invite participants to stay online for any information discussion that you would like to host. Make a little quiet time for yourself after the meeting to reflect on what did and did not work well at the meeting and to consider how you can make future video meetings (even) better. Get up, walk about and stop thinking about work for a short while – before the next video meeting.

Key Points

- In preparing for a video meeting, consider the following issues: who, what, where, when, why
- If you are the host, anticipate everything that can go wrong and try to prevent or mitigate these problems
- If you are presenting at the meeting, check in advance what facilities you will have, for example, to activate your microphone, to share slides on the screen, and to see incoming chat comments or questions
- Because of variable quality of internet connections, tend to speak slowly, clearly and briefly
- Without the quality of nonverbal communication possible at in-person meetings, be careful in any use of humour, sarcasm or irony in video meetings
- For participants at the meeting, be sure you understand the protocols and etiquette in terms of having your camera on or off, muting microphone, raising 'hands', or making verbal or written comments. Assume that your microphone is live unless you check that it is off.

Practical Exercise

Send a Zoom invitation to all members of the teaching group and the teachers for a 10-minute meeting. The teachers use the session to give a 10-minute talk about how to take part in a video meeting. The students are given no other instructions except for the login details. The Zoom meeting is, with participants' approval, recorded.

After the video meeting, the students return to the table in the meeting room. The teacher then continues to complete the talk about how to take part in a Zoom meeting in a live session.

Then the 10-minute video of the meeting is played back. Using a stop-start technique, the teacher invites comments from the group at key learning points. After showing the whole video, the teacher further summarises comments. The video of the 10-minute meeting is then played to the whole group.

A final part of the session consists of a further 10-minute video meeting in which each member of the group is asked what they have learned from the session. The teachers summarise at the end what has improved between the first and second videos.

CHAPTER 20

How to Present a Proposal for Funding

If you apply for funding for a research or service project, very often this is a fully written process, with either one or two stages in the application before you hear if your application is successful. But sometimes the funding body will ask you to attend for an interview, if you are shortlisted. This chapter offers information about preparing for such an interview and what to do at such a meeting.

RELATED CHAPTERS

Chapter 18. How to behave in an interview for a post
Chapter 21. How to make an elevator pitch
Chapter 29. How to convince others of the usefulness of a project

Preparation for the Meeting

Read the invitation to the application meeting very carefully. Check if you are invited to or are told to make an **initial presentation** at the meeting, for example, summarising your proposal. Check the details carefully. Can you use slides? What is the maximum time allowed for the presentation? Is the number of slides specified? Does the funder tell you what issues to address in the presentation? The group of applicants need to draft and redraft this presentation over as long as possible before the actual interview day. Ask friendly but critical colleagues to join you for **practice rehearsals** and to give you critical and constructive feedback. Be sure that your presentation is no longer than the given **time limit**. There will often be a limit to how many of your team can attend the interview, so try to select staff who are both very good communicators and represent different disciplines, backgrounds or perspectives, to have a **strong, complementary team**. Thus, for example, if your proposal deals with doing some work in the community, include a representative of the community in the group that will make the presentation.

Remember also to **introduce those who will join you** to make a presentation of your proposal by highlighting their particular skills or relevant experience. When asked a question, try to involve those accompanying you in answering it.

When answering questions – and in making your presentation – think of who will read it and what their expertise, prejudices, preferences and obligations might be.

Anticipate and Prepare Probable Questions

Arrange for your group of applicants to meet and to **anticipate questions** likely to be asked at the interview. For each probable question, develop an outline for the agreed response, as you prepare. If a group of applicants attend the interview, agree in advance **who will answer** each question. Ensure that the members of your team have several questions they are ready to answer. Ask your critical colleagues to **identify weaknesses** in the application. Expect to be asked about these at the interview.

If your proposal has been through a **peer review** process, and if you have the reports of the peer reviewers, expect that any or all of the problems identified by the reviewers will be explored during the interview. Prepare detailed replies to each issue and decide before the interview if you want to change any aspects of your proposal in response to reviewers' comments. Try to find out from the funding organisation who the panel members are. Prepare a **short biographical note** about each panel member for your application team. For each panel member, think in advance about **what their probable perspective is** on the application. What are they likely to see as the hallmarks of a very strong application? Prepare to be able to favourably comment a little on the important work of each panel member, without overexaggerating this form of flattery.

Mock Interviews

If the award you have applied for is large or is very important to you, arrange two or three 'dress rehearsals'. At these practice meetings, ask senior colleagues to play the part of the interview panel members, and arrange for the whole group of applicants who will later go to the real interview, to attend. Ask the mock panel members to be fairly **hard in their questions**. Ideally the mock interview will be tougher than the real thing. Have a colleague sitting to one side at the meeting to take notes about the performance of your team and the feedback from the panel. Identify a coordinator for your applicant group to direct particular questions to specific members of your group, ensuring that **all members have the chance to substantially contribute** to the discussion.

Often the **format for a dress rehearsal** is as follows: (1) the chair of the panel welcomes the group of applicants; (2) the applicants make a 5–10-minute presentation summarising the application; (3) the panel members each ask the applicant two or three questions; (4) after the role play part of the meeting the chair may ask the applicants for their views of their performance; and (5) the chair asks each member of the interview panel to give positive and negative feedback points to the applicants (during this time is it helpful for the applicants to be silent and not to make defensive comments). To **conclude the meeting**, the lead person for the applicants usually offers thanks to the mock interview panel for their time and constructive support. Allow at least a week between a series of mock interviews to give your group of applicants time to refine and improve their performance. Before the interview day, **send your slides** to the funding body and ask for confirmation that they have safely received them. Agree your **central core messages** with your applicant group before the meeting. Simplify and refine these and make sure that you are ready to include these messages in the live interview, even if this means stating these when they are not directly relevant to the questions asked, by forging links or bridges from the questions to your key points.

If you will not have an opportunity to show slides, prepare the description of your proposal in a small series of paper posters (in A4 format) – one containing only the title and possibly another sentence; one listing the individual who is going to be the team, indicating – by underlining or bolding – who is accompanying you as a presenter. You might add a few more sheets of paper, each with no more than a paragraph or two – imitating a slideshow – with the description of the goals, the method, the timing and the budget. Make sure that the paper is of good quality and make sufficient copies for the members of the committee. You should keep a copy of this proposal but the members of the team should not – it should be obvious that they know the project by heart.

Starting the Interview

At the actual interview, **arrive early** and make time to relax as much as possible. **Dress formally**. If you are not the first group of applicants to be interviewed, expect to start later than your given time, as many factors can cause delays in the interview schedule. As you are **invited into the interview room**, wait for the panel chair to invite you to sit. Do not go forward to shake hands or otherwise greet the panel members unless they invite you to. Try to arrange for your coordinator to sit in the middle of your group. Briefly **introduce each member** of your group to the panel, indicating their speciality. When invited to, start your introductory presentation.

Key Issues to Emphasise During the Presentation and Question Period

Keep in mind the following key issues during the presentation and question and answer session:

- Make a clear **summary** statement about your main proposal at or near the start of the meeting.
- State your **central key messages** at the start of the meeting and again at the end.
- Say why this work is **important**, and to whom it is important.
- In the short term, who will **benefit**?
- What are the **implications** of this work in the long-term, and how many people may benefit and how?
- What are the risks – for the donors, the subject, the programme – and how are they neutralised?

- What is your **track record** in this area?
- During your answers, stress the different skills and perspectives of your team, and how this **multidisciplinarity** is a strength of your proposal.
- How much have you **consulted** with groups who may be affected by your proposed work?
- Have you established **partnerships** with groups who can strengthen your project, or who can harm or stop your project if they are not happy with the plans? Consider whether you can invite one of those who will be affected by the project's execution or results to join the presenting team.
- If you are awarded the funding for the project, who will **benefit financially**, and when and how?
- In the project period, how many **participants** will there be, and where will they be?
- What is the **budget** and how is it allocated?
- What is the **timeline** for the whole project and for its component parts or phases?
- How will the **impact** of the project be assessed and by whom?
- What are the intended deliverables, benefits or outcomes?
- If you have described stages or **phases** of your project, refer to these clearly and consistently and add a few brief words about each phase so that the panel members are fully orientated to the components of your project and their time sequence.

During your presentation, keep in mind the needs of the members of the panel and try to offer some gain or **benefit to each panel member** or their constituency. For example, if the project will take place in a particular town or neighbourhood, will some local organisations there gain funding? If the project will be conducted in a hospital or clinic, will staff and patients be financially reimbursed for their time and contributions?

After the Interview

You and your team may be emotionally fatigued by the stress of the interview. Congratulate everyone on their contributions. Give yourself time to **relax and deescalate** – perhaps find a café. There is no need to have a detailed debriefing immediately – arrange for feedback within the group over the following few days. Think about what went well and what did not go so well. If possible, **seek feedback** from those present (committee or other staff) on your presentation and performance. If possible, seek written feedback from the committee on the interview. From this feedback, see if you can make your next funding interview even stronger.

Key Points

- It is vital to practice presenting your proposal before the real event
- For important awards or grants, have several formal practice events
- Seek feedback from your mock interviews and identify your weaknesses
- Anticipate the most likely questions and prepare detailed answers
- Select your team for the presentation carefully for people who can speak well and persuasively in public and who represent the range of stakeholders in your group
- Distribute your speaking time relatively equally among your group members
- Have a group coordinator who manages who will answer which questions
- If you need to make an initial presentation, for example, with slides, revise and refine these carefully to make sure that your main points are communicated clearly
- Take the interview seriously, dress formally and arrive early
- Identify before the interview who the panel members are, and in your presentation aim to offer benefits to each of them and their constituencies

Practical Exercise

At least a day or two before the session on presenting the proposal, the teacher divides the whole student group into subgroups, each with about five or six members. The task is to prepare and present a proposal for a special grant of 100,000 euros for a project. Each group has to prepare an 8-minute presentation in which they will summarise their proposal. During the session, all the students see all the presentations. The selection panel consists of the local hospital director, a senior person in the Ministry of Health, and a senior leader from the local community. After each presentation, the panel members ask each team questions about their proposal for about 10 minutes. After the interviews have taken place, the students watch as the panel members discuss the strengths and weaknesses of each of the three proposals. Finally, the panel decides which, if any, of the three proposal teams will win the special 100,000 euro award. There is a brief final discussion for the whole group.

CHAPTER 21

How to Make an Elevator Pitch

From time to time, you may have an idea that you really want to put into practice. Some of these you can simply implement yourself. But others will require resources that are beyond your immediate command. In this case you will need to try to **persuade people who do have these resources to invest in you** and your idea. One opportunity for such persuasion is when you can contact an influential person for a brief discussion, during which time you summarise your proposal. Unless you deliberately arrange them, these opportunities arise rarely and unpredictably, for example, coming across such a 'gateway' person in an elevator or lift. These chances are therefore called 'the elevator pitch'. In this chapter we offer information on how to prepare, deliver and follow up on such pitches. Related chapters are shown below.

> **RELATED CHAPTERS**
>
> Chapter 6. How to behave in an interview with the media
> Chapter 15. How to write a report of a meeting
> Chapter 18. How to behave in an interview for a post
> Chapter 20. How to present a proposal for funding
> Chapter 29. How to convince others of the usefulness of a project

Preparation

The task is to prepare a short statement of about **a minute or less** (about 50–200 words) summarising your proposal and why the other person (whom we call here 'the target' of the pitch) should be interested in it. Because such a chance can occurring without any warning, you need to be able to present your idea clearly, briefly and persuasively at any time, for example, to a wealthy philanthropist or to a governmental minister. Preparation is therefore vital.

As you begin drafting your own notes for your pitch, identify **what you want to achieve** from a pitch meeting. You will not secure any clear agreement or undertaking from the target. The most realistic aim is that your target pitch expresses some, if limited, interest in your idea at the initial meeting and then invites you to **send in further details** to their office, or perhaps to meet with their staff. You cannot expect a direct meeting with the target or their staff at this early stage. What you do need to do is to have a **personal card ready**, with your contact details, to give to your target and to their assistant.

Your pitch will need to contain several very short segments in which you summarise, in a few sentences, your core message. The **five Ws framework** presented in Chapter 15 is one way to get straight to the point, for example, using these components:

- Who are you?
- What do you want to do?
- Where do you want to do it and when?
- Why is this important?
- What is the next step?

WHO ARE YOU?

Say, in a few words, enough to place you in the imagination of the target. Where do you work, what is your role, and **what experience** do you have? Be specific. Try to include at least one memorable and **unusual characteristic** about yourself.

WHAT DO YOU WANT TO DO?

Be very brief in giving the target and their entourage a **short version of your project or proposal**. Cut out all details. Say who and **how many people will benefit**, and how visible this benefit will be.

WHERE DO YOU WANT TO DO IT AND WHEN?

Summarise **where and when** the project will take place. Be sure that the work is within the responsibilities of the target. Try to **connect and align what you want to do with their current interests**, priorities or investments. Show your target that you are very familiar with their work and how impressed you are with their achievements.

WHY IS THIS PROJECT IMPORTANT?

In emphatic and perhaps even emotional terms, explain why this work is **vital and urgent**. What is the need or challenge to be addressed or remedied? You may want to describe this as the problem and the solution. What is your answer to this challenge and why is it interesting and effective? Why are you **sure that your approach will work**? What benefit will the project bring to the target? What **positive publicity or profile** can they gain from supporting your idea. When will the benefit be realised? If you can, think of a **memorable phrase or 'hook'** that will make your target remember what you have said.

WHAT IS THE NEXT STEP?

This is sometimes termed the **'call to action'**. What do you want to happen next? A meeting? For them to open an email you will send to them and to reply to you? **Be specific** in your request.

REHEARSE AND PRACTICE

As we emphasise in many other chapters of this book, preparation and practice are essential for success. Your first draft pitch is very likely to be **too long and too boring**. Find a willing colleague, friend or family member to help you. Do not read your pitch but **speak it aloud**. Do not use notes or prompts. Time how long it takes. If you can, **audio- or videotape** these rehearsals and subject yourself to the possibly embarrassing rigours of replaying your performance. Remember, you are aiming for 1—2 minutes only. Ask for **frank feedback** about what is not clear or what is not interesting in what you say. Ask your commentator if they would invest in this idea or not and why. In some countries there are television shows, such as The Apprentice, which are centred upon a pitch for a business idea that tries to persuade a sceptical panel of experts to invest. Watch these shows and learn from how the contestants pitch.

After drafting the initial pitch, **refine your briefing notes** to yourself and then rehearse again, and again. Cut out everything that is not essential. Tend to use short and strong words, especially active verbs. Use **confident phrases** such as 'I firmly believe…' or 'I am confident that…'. Remember that the elevator pitch is not only selling your idea, but also at least as much about **selling yourself**. As you go live you are likely to feel nervous, and for many people one effect of feeling tense is to flatten the emotional tone of how they look and speak. To compensate for this, **overemphasise your enthusiasm** as you speak – your commentator will tell you if you overdo it!

Delivering the Pitch Live

Opportunities to pitch can occur by serendipity, such as unexpectedly actually sharing a lift or elevator with your target, or can **happen with some planning** on your part. For example, you may attend a conference, seminar or round table where your target features, and you can try to find a short time after the meeting to introduce yourself and make your statement. Or you can see that your target will be present at a meal during a high-profile meeting, and you can seek a moment when they do not have official duties, for example, over initial drinks, to make your move. Your target is likely to be either an influential or an affluent person, so dress formally in the style of others at the meeting. Greet the person or their assistant and **ask if you can have a moment** of their time. Be prepared for the answer to be no. Such people are pitched or propositioned all the time. They know that an approach will probably be from a person wanting something from them. If you do have a positive response, plunge straight in.

Give your pitch with **confidence and conviction**, and smile while you speak. Have your personal calling card ready. As you finish, say you would be happy to provide further details or to meet to take the idea further. Try hard to **appear pleasant** and to be the type of person they would like to do business with. Especially, because you have so little time, speak **clearly and slowly**. Give stress and emphasis to your most important words and ideas. Do not forget to breathe! Do not rush and try to pack in more content. Establish and keep strong **eye contact** with your target. Be **flexible**. If the initial response links your idea to another programme, say how positive you are about the opportunity.

After the Pitch

Making a pitch is a high energy and high stakes situation. Prepare to be gently, firmly or rudely declined or rejected. You may need to make many pitches before you receive any expression of interest. Find a **quite spot to relax** and reflect. Consider what went well or less well during the pitch. Check to see if they gave you any encouragement for follow-up or not. If not, do not contact the target or their staff. If there was a clear interest, or a mixed message, **send a short written version** (one page or less) of your proposal to the contact person within the next 24 hours, pointing out when and where you met, and saying you would be very happy to provide further details.

Key Points

- Prepare your pitch very carefully, for example, giving the five Ws: Who are you? What do you want to do? Where do you want to do it and when? Why do your project?
- Rehearse your pitch many times, to cut it down to 1 minute or less, speaking without notes
- Ask for and listen to advice and feedback about your draft pitches
- Make your presentation compelling, and full of confidence and conviction
- Introduce yourself very briefly with at least one memorable characteristic about yourself
- Try to identify occasions when you can meet your pitch target, for example, on the fringes of formal meetings
- Whether or not your pitch leads to further contact with your target, reflect on how to pitch better in future

Practical Exercise

The aim of this practical exercise is to learn how to make an elevator pitch by practising this skill. This exercise is a simulation of the situation in which you, for example, by accident, meet your target person in a lift/elevator (such as a minister of health) and you have about a minute to present ('pitch') your proposal. When making a presentation, it might be effective to start by the statement that summarises it.

Each member of the group is invited to prepare a 1-minute statement to summarise a proposal that is important to them. Spend 10–15 minutes preparing your proposal. A smaller number, for example, four or five students, are then asked to stand up one at a time and deliver their pitch. After all the pitches, the whole group comments and offers feedback on the more and the less effective pitches. Feedback should be specific about what works well and what could be improved. The presenters should listen to the feedback without responding or defending their presentation. At the end, the teacher(s) summarise key learning points, which can include the following:

Each 1-minute pitch should include:

- Identify *what* your plan/proposal is (be as specific as you can)
- Clarify *why* this is important
- Say *how* this helps the person you are presenting your idea to (e.g., to achieve their aims)
- Very briefly say how long this project would take and *when* results will be available
- Spell out what are the *next steps* that need to be taken

CHAPTER 22

How to Negotiate

The ability to negotiate can be invaluable to you in many aspects of your life. In this chapter, we focus upon practical skills that can help you to negotiate and to achieve, or partly achieve, your goals in the work setting. Related chapters are shown below.

Th origin of 'negotiate' stems from the Latin word *negotiatus,* meaning 'to carry on business, do business', and is a combination of the terms *neg*, meaning not, and *otium*, meaning leisure. Over about the last 500 years, the English use of the word has evolved to mean **to communicate with one or more other people in search of a mutual agreement**.

Preparing to Negotiate

As we mentioned in Chapter 18, when taking part in an interview, **preparation is a vital aspect** of using this skill. Decide from the very start of your preparation what your **minimum acceptable end point** is. This means the point at which you will discontinue the negotiation without reaching an agreement. If the negotiations involve several people, find out about them in detail, both those on your side and on the other side. A negotiation is essentially about a **conflict of needs or interests**. You will be trying to reach a point at which **both sides can accept a less than optimal solution** and come away from the discussion with self-esteem and pride intact. In this case, a large part of the preparation for a negotiation must focus on a detailed **understanding of what the other side needs** to achieve and why they want to achieve this, and on anticipating their probably minimally acceptable solution. In short, you need to put yourself in their shoes and to **understand their point of view**. From this perspective, it can also be important to find out what other items might be of interest to the team with which you negotiate: perhaps you can make the others accept a less than ideal solution from their point of view if you offer some benefits unrelated to the item that is the subject of negotiation.

Get as much information about the **track record of negotiation by the other side**. If the discussion simply involves one other person, for example, you want your manager to increase your salary, find out if you can what has happened when other colleagues made this proposal to this manager or to other managers in the organisation. Make a **list of precedents that strengthen your argument** or your proposal.

If you are part of a negotiating team, prepare carefully **what each team member will do**, and when and how. Agree who will speak first and what opening position you will take – how much or how little will you say about your demands early in the negotiation? Will you all give exactly the same messages to the other side, or will you deliberately give somewhat conflicting proposals, to disorientate the opposition? Whatever your approach, fundamentally, **your team must be clear, unified and disciplined**. If any member of your team is not committed to the agreed 'line to take', they need to be dropped from the team, even if this occurs at short notice when no replacement is possible. It is important that the members of your team do not surprise you by approaches, offers or comments. To avoid this, it is helpful to have relatively **frequent breaks in the negotiations**, to consider new ideas that team members might have before putting them onto the negotiation table.

Plan to conduct every step of the negotiation in a **respectful and courteous** way (see also similarities in Chapter 23 on How to say No). Maintain a **neutral emotional tone**. Whatever provocation you may encounter, do not become angry.

During the Negotiation

Start with introductions of all participants and note the seniority of your counterparts. Beware of any member of the other team arriving late without an introduction. During the opening remarks, try to delay making any specific proposals, to **allow the opportunity for the other side to be the first with concrete proposals**. When you do make your first proposal on the topic of the negotiation, **overstate or overbid as your initial offer**. This needs careful judgement. How far should one overstate the initial proposal? How many details can be sacrificed for the sake of agreement later? What is the value of each negotiating point? Can you find concessions that are of less value to you and of more value to the other side? Thus for your side it might be unimportant what name the project will have, whereas the other group may be very keen to have a project carry a particular name. Do not give up such points that are of no importance to your side: the value for the other team should be taken into account.

Then see if both sides are willing and able to make a **series of small concessions** towards closing the gap between their starting points. Less experienced negotiators tend to make concessions that are too large at each step. Note if there is a **symmetry in the pattern of concessions**, for example, your reducing your main proposal by 5% in each discussion round and whether the other side makes a similar proportionate reduction in their demands. If concessions are asymmetrical you may want to state this openly. **Only trade something for something** – do not make a concession unless the other side also does the same. **Only make conditional offers**. Say what you can do to enhance your offer, depending on specific improvements that you need to see from the other side.

If the issue being negotiated is important to you and you are conducting the negotiation alone, try to arrange for an **advisor or supporter to be available** for the whole time allocated for the meeting. At any time you can call for a break in the negotiations so that your team, or you and your advisor, can find a confidential place to take stock of the nature of the discussion, and decide whether to maintain your agreed approach on strategy and tactics, or whether to adapt by changing either.

If the **other side makes a statement that you know to be untrue, interrupt and neutralise this point immediately**. If any statement by the other side is not clear, **ask them to make this clear** straight away. Make notes during the meeting, or, if this is agreed, record the meeting. During the discussion do not make any assumptions about what the other side wants. Use clarifying questions as much as you need to, to make what they want clearer to you.

Support or **bolster your proposals with strong points**. These can be relevant statistics, survey results, patient or consumer statements, or indications of your track record. Only speak of your own capabilities positively. Try to show relentlessly that you are seeking an agreement that **both sides can report as a 'win'**. The other side will also likely state their main strengths. Do not hesitate to correct these if their statements are incorrect or exaggerated, but do this politely. As the discussion proceeds, have a series of staged strong points or tokens in reserve, which you can add into the balance at key points to try to trigger greater concessions from the other side. Do not say at any stage what your 'bottom line' or minimum acceptable position would be. Towards the end of the meeting try to **introduce additional elements** that you want to capture, especially assets that you know are highly valuable to you but not so valuable to the other side. It is of great importance to establish the ranking of proposals of the other side. Find out what is of particular importance to them and build your strategy taking this into account.

If you find that the other side is **behaving aggressively or disrespectfully**, you have several options. You can use contrasting styles: if they are loud you can speak quietly; if they speak quickly and try to rush you, you can speak rather slowly. If they interrupt you, give way each time and then pause for a few seconds each time they finish. Do not state or imply blame. Ignore all threats. Demonstrate a confident and patient firmness of purpose.

If the discussion moves to an offer that you would find acceptable, **do not accept too soon**. You may find that further arguments on your side will lead to an even better offer. Maintain a positive tone to the discussion and praise the other side for their fairness and flexibility. Beware late surprises. One tactic is for a team to keep in reserve a critical asset that they want to gain, and to not even **mention this until very late in the day**, when you may be tired or short of time. To try to prevent this, it is usually helpful to ask the opposition at the start of the meeting to list all the variables or assets that can be included in the discussion, and for details of any issues that cannot be included in the negotiation. At a late stage of the discussion, if you are not sure whether to settle for an agreement or not, you can call for a brief break for you to consult a 'senior colleague', who may or may not exist! It is also important that your negotiating team does not have two leaders. If no compromise about the seniority can be found, do not include one of the leaders in your team.

Successful negotiations will very often leave **both sides having achieved some, but not all, of their objectives**. If an agreement is reached, make positive remarks on a highly successful meeting, give a **detailed summary of your understanding of what has been agreed**, and ask the other side to say whether this is a full and fair precis of the agreement. Keep a clear focus on your minimally acceptable position. If this is not reached, simply say so, giving the other side some time to move further towards what you want to achieve. If they do not, then pause or stop the negotiation, expressing disappointment that agreement has not been reached, remaining polite throughout. Decide before the meeting that if you do reach this point, will you declare that the negotiation has ended or will you leave open the door to a potential future further round of negotiation?

After the Negotiation Meeting

As is the case for many other important meetings (see Chapter 15 on How to write a report of a meeting), if there is not a **written record** of the discussion then, in a sense, the meeting did not take place. Take the initiative and draft a detailed summary of the meeting, focusing especially on what specifically was agreed, and who will do what as a consequence of the agreement and over what timescale. Be as specific as you can, to leave as little room for ambiguity or misunderstanding as possible in your summary. Send this as a **draft summary** to the other team and ask for any corrections to this summary as a fair record of the agreement, giving them a relatively short timescale to reply. After their reply, aim to finalise the agreement quickly with **details of how it will be implemented**. Throughout all stages of the negotiation, focus on your aims of concluding this negotiation successfully and maintaining good relationships to allow further business dealings with your counterpart in future.

Key Points

- Preparation is absolutely vital for a successful negotiation
- Decide in advance what your minimum or maximum acceptable outcomes of the negotiation are
- Put yourself in the shoes of your opposite number and try to find out and understand what they want from the negotiation and what value they are likely to attach to your possible concessions
- Get background information on the members of the opponent's team
- Plan what each member of your team will do and when. Agree on your approach and what your group is and is not willing to negotiate upon
- Try to arrange for the other side to make the initial proposals for a deal or a compromise, then make minor concessions and wait to see if the other side does the same

- See if there is a symmetry in the pattern of the concessions or not
- Support your proposals and concessions with strong statements
- If the other side makes incorrect statements, correct them at once
- Tend to behave courteously and respectfully unless the other side is consistently rude or aggressive
- Record each step of the negotiation
- If a tentative agreement is reached, summarise or paraphrase it and check that both sides agree to the same wording
- Note that successful negotiations will very often leave both sides having achieved some, but not all, of their objectives, and with the relationship intact ready for future meetings or negotiations.

Additional Resources

Kennedy, G. (2008). The pocket negotiator. London: The Economist Books.

CHAPTER 23

How to Say No

For many staff, there is a fine line between having a manageable amount of work to do (and to try to do well) and simply having too much work to do. In many roles the majority of tasks are obligatory, for example, direct patient care for doctors. But often there are categories of work that are discretionary. In Chapter 41 we discuss how to decide on your priorities in your life. There we discuss making time periodically to assess which tasks before you are urgent or important, and which ones are not, and to allocate your time accordingly. Another way to try to gain control over your work and time is to develop the ability to say No. Related chapters are shown below.

RELATED CHAPTERS

Chapter 22. How to negotiate
Chapter 24. How to manage a poorly performing colleague
Chapter 26. How to reduce tension in a small group or in a meeting
Chapter 42. How to admit an error or apologise

When invited to take on a task that is not obligatory for you, there are several **reasons why you may be tempted to say yes**. If you are in a junior position, the invitation may well come from your manager or senior, and you will want to create a good impression in their eyes. In a system of patronage, such as most health care professions, you may feel that you need to accept all your manager's offers to increase the likelihood that they will help you with your future career. The invitation may be to do something that you find unusual, interesting or important. But if you accept all the invitations to take on extra or discretionary work, you are likely to become overwhelmed very soon, so that you cannot do any of your work well, and this will probably leave you feeling guilty, fatigued and demoralised. So, how do you say No? We suggest the following approach to declining invitations.

First, show great **courtesy and politeness** to the person asking you to perform this extra task. It is possible that they simply want to dump you with the work, but it is also possible that they hold you in high esteem, are impressed by your accomplishments, and expect that you can do this task well. Whatever the reason for the invitation, treat the other person very kindly.

Next, **summarise what you understand the task to be**. Give a brief but fairly detailed summary of this role or challenge, and show that you have carefully considered accepting the invitation. Demonstrate that you are a thoughtful person who tries to take decisions carefully and responsibly.

Then, go on to make some **counterproposals**, if you can. For example, you may wish to say that you can perform this suggested work, but within the next 6 months, not 3 months. Or you may say that your expertise or experience does not extend to the whole undertaking, but that you can take on doing the first part of a three-part task. You may also wish to **negotiate on resources**. For example, you may say that you already have a rather full workload, but that you could contribute about a quarter of the work required if other colleagues are also allocated to contribute. If possible, suggest particular people who you would like to work with, and get their agreement before proposing them.

Another tactic is to **bargain about the offer**. One option is to say that you may be able to take on the new tasks if some part of your current workload is taken away. Or you may ask, for example, for an extra week of leave in the following summer if you take on the new role. You may ask for a block of additional time for your holidays, or to count the days of additional work you dedicate to the task and agree before starting that you can take the equivalent amount of time off in lieu (often called TOIL) at a later date. A variant of this approach is to **calculate how much you are normally paid** for each day of your usual work, and to seek agreement at the outset that you will be given extra pay later on, calculated on the basis of the number of extra days of work you undertake, which may be an accumulated total of additional work you do during evenings and weekends. If you choose to negotiate, then make it easy for the other person to engage. You can make several counter proposals and ask the other person for their views on which may be feasible.

Next, we consider the case where **you really do not want to take on the additional task**. If you decide to decline the invitation, we suggest you reply to the invitation very soon to say so, and then the more senior person may still have time to find someone else to take on the role. When you decline, first say that it was an honour to have received this invitation. Say that unfortunately you do not have the necessary skills, if this is true. You could go on to say that as you are not skilled in this area, you would not want your efforts to damage the reputation of your department.

If you can, bring a possible solution to the challenge. For example, you may propose another person for the work, if you have their agreement. Usually, senior staff have a much more positive view of junior staff who give them not just a problem (a refusal to do the extra work), but also a solution.

If you do need to **completely decline the invitation**, try to break this bad news gently to the other person. You can say, for example, that you are honoured or humbled to be invited to be involved in this very important type of work. State that under normal circumstances you would be delighted to accept the invitation, but that you reluctantly need to reply by saying that you are not able to accept. Try to avoid giving a short and straight No. Do not simply say that you do not have enough time to do the extra work. Most people you work with will feel that they do not have enough time in the day to meet all their expectations. In your reply, indicate how much you value the relationship you have with the other person. If you wish to give a reason for declining, for example, that you have an important examination coming soon, then give only one reason, not more than one – do not protest too much. Be sincere in what you say, and only give true reasons why you cannot accept. In your reply, try hard to ensure that in saying No, you maintain, as far as you can, a good working relationship with your senior colleague, perhaps by saying that you hope that circumstances will allow you to accept invitations for additional work in the future.

If your working situation is one where power relationships, and perhaps a **patronage system** of career advancement, mean that you cannot refuse invitations from your manager, perhaps find some positive aspect in this by noting down in your journal or your diary these events, and what you will learn from them to guide you when you become a manager or leader in the future, either by copying your own manager's behaviour, or by doing the opposite yourself when you are in a position of responsibility.

Further points to keep in mind when saying No have been described by Zoe Williams in the British newspaper *The Guardian* (13th December 2023), and can include the following:

- Vary how direct or detailed your refusal is, according to the strength of your relationship with the person.
- Have a graded response, for example, 'I can do this on this occasion, but next time I need more notice'.
- If you say No, you need to mean it and maintain your No – no backsliding.
- Try to say No to a particular proposal and make it emotionally neutral – do not criticise the person who produced the idea.
- Renegotiate the offer – if it is to meet at 7 a.m., perhaps say you could meet at 9 a.m. or 10 a.m.
- Stop and think to consider invitations carefully and ask yourself, 'If this were happening tomorrow and not next month, would I accept?'.
- If you need to decline an invitation and this may upset the other person, do it early and not late.
- If you are unsure about a proposal, say you need time to reflect upon it.
- If you do not have time for a new and interesting task, ask your colleague if there is another task you can drop to allow you to do the new work.
- On some occasions you may not want to give a complete refusal, and you can say 'My current commitments mean that unfortunately I'm not able to take this on now, but perhaps we can discuss it again next [week/month/year]'.
- Remember the golden rule: treat other people as you would want to be treated yourself, when – for whatever reason – you choose to say No.

Practical Exercise

Four members of a group are identified to issue invitations for these four situations to take place one week in the future:

1. A patient invites a doctor to a meal at the patient's home.
2. A senior person invites a junior person to a meal.

3. A junior person invites a senior person to a meal.

4. A political party not supported by a junior member of staff invites that staff member to give a talk in support of the party at a political meeting.

Four more members of the teaching group are identified – one each to respond to one of these invitations. In the practical exercise, the first invitation is presented orally and the first invitee gives an oral negative response. These is repeated for invitations two, three and four.

Next the four interviewees are invited to say how they felt when declining their invitation. The whole group is invited to comment on all four examples of saying No. The teachers ask the group to comment on (1) whether the declines were given as they should be given, and (2) how else the decliners could have said No. Finally, the teachers make summarising comments about ways to say No that may include the following points:

- Whether accepting or declining the invitation, try to act so that the relationship with the person issuing the invitation is maintained.
- Take all invitations seriously as they may have serious consequences.
- Decide if you wish to give a reason for saying No, or not. Do not give too many reasons.
- Truthfulness is important, as is politeness.
- Decide if you want to decline that particular time and date of an invitation or to decline any meeting at all.
- Declining an invitation completely is perhaps the most difficult situation and if you say No completely, be aware that you may need to accept the consequences of this decision.

CHAPTER 24

How to Manage a Poorly Performing Colleague

A great deal of the work carried out by health and care staff, as well as by researchers, takes place in teams. Within teams there may be colleagues who at times do not carry out their work very well. This may be because they are not capable of performing their role, or because they are capable but have reasons not to undertake the work properly. Whether or not you are responsible for such a colleague, you may find that you need to know how to deal with a poorly performing colleague. This chapter offers options on how to address this common challenge. Related chapters are shown below.

The Poorly Performing Colleague Who Is a Peer

If you are involved in trying to assist such a colleague, we suggest that you first of all **define what role you play**. If you are a direct colleague of equal status in your organisation, you can play a supporting role by spending time talking to the colleague. Decide if you will offer advice. If you do offer advice, you may be disappointed if this is not taken. If your advice is taken and is not successful, you may be blamed by the individual. A **constructive discussion** does not need to involve you giving advice. You can **listen to the person** and try to understand their situation. You can ask what options they have tried to improve their situation. You can ask what further possibilities the person can envisage to make an improvement, and then ask what the **advantages and disadvantages for each course of action** are. You can go further and ask about what is stopping the person from taking a decision or acting upon their decisions.

In the process of such a discussion, try to **understand that person's situation** and the challenges they face. Is the job too demanding or not demanding enough? Is the relationship with the manager supportive or undermining? Are they still learning and acquiring new skills or feeling bored and demoralised? What is the **home and family background**? Are relationships at home on a strong or weak footing? Has there been a recent loss or bereavement? Are family unwell and far away? Are there severe or deteriorating financial pressures? The problems you see in the work performance of the colleague may have their **origins outside the workplace**.

Is the person going through a period of **stress or burnout**, or mental ill health? Can you create a confidential atmosphere or **'safe space'** so that the person feels able to disclose such difficulties? Mental health problems are common in the general population and especially common among health and care staff, but stigma can make talking about this difficult or impossible. Do you have the impression that mental health problems are severe or that the person needs immediate assistance? Will they seek help? Will they accept you making a referral or accompanying them to an assessment?

Is there any form of **physical illness or disability** that limits the person's ability to carry out their work role, and has this been recognised by the employer? Are any forms of assistance or adjustments being provided to support the person to succeed in their role? If you did meet your colleague in the role of a peer offering support, try to show concern and compassion, but try to remain objective and not to become emotionally overinvolved with their difficulties. Be cautious in case the person is sharing their problems with very many people and is receiving a great deal of conflicting advice. For such informal contact, offer to meet again and to keep in touch, at a frequency you can manage. Decide if you do or do not want to offer that the person can contact you directly, for example, by phone or text message.

The Poorly Performing Colleague Who You Manage

If you are in the position of the manager of the person whose work falls below the required standard, your situation is very different from that of a colleague or peer. Before initiating contact with the colleague, we suggest that you become very **familiar with the relevant procedures** of your organisation. Possibly with different wording, these will probably refer to *capability* (whether the person is capable of performing a particular work role to the expected standard) and *conduct* (meaning that the person is capable of working to the required standard, but for some reason is not doing so). To learn or remind yourself what the workplace procedures are, you can consult the organisation's human resources policy or ask colleagues in that department to brief you.

In many organisations, there are two stages in managing the poorly performing colleague: the **informal stage and the formal stage**. At the earlier informal stage, you will probably need to:

- Inform the person in writing that you want to arrange a meeting to discuss their work performance

- Indicate that you would like to discuss the situation and aim to come to a mutual agreement on what steps to take to resolve the issues
- Say if the person can bring a supporter or representative (such as from a trade union or syndicate) to the meeting or not

At the initial **informal meeting**, as the manager you will most probably want to:

- Try to put the person at their ease
- Be specific about what aspects of their work are not adequate
- Not say what your sources of information are, if there has been a confidential complaint from another colleague
- Say that the meeting is a part of an informal procedure, according to the policy of the organisation
- Say that you will make a note of the meeting and share this after the meeting, to have an agreed record of what was said and agreed

We suggest that after this initial setting of the scene, you focus on **listening**. Ask how the person sees the situation. Note what the person says and also how they say it and their emotional tone. Do they accept that there is a problem or not? Do they seem to want assistance? Do you feel that the person is giving a full account of the problems? Try very hard to be nonjudgemental. Avoid blame. Try to create an approach that is one of joint problem solving. As for a peer, try to understand that person's life situation, predicament, pressures and dilemmas. Put yourself in their shoes.

After the listening phase, move on to **identifying possible actions** as remedies. Ask the person for their suggestions about who can do what to make improvements. Test each idea to see if it is feasible. Put possible actions into a sequence and a timeframe. Agree on a plan of action and set a date for a second meeting to review if these actions are leading to improvements in work performance. Before the second meeting, try to agree the record of the meeting with your colleague, and use the agreed action plan, as specifically as possible, as the basis for subsequent discussions.

Before subsequent meetings, **gather objective data** on whether the person's work is improving, using specific ways to assess this and avoiding any general critical comments that may be unfair or discriminatory towards that person. If the plan is not producing benefits in the workplace, ask for further suggestions from the person. Try to get an impression about whether there may be underlying problems that have not been disclosed, for example, alcohol or drug use, marital tensions, or severe fatigue or insomnia.

As the manager, try to be aware that in dealing with an underperforming colleague **you are working both for that person, but also for the benefit of the work team**. An incompetent or poorly motivated colleague can be a toxic element within a team, especially where the consequence is more work for other team members. This will be seen as unfair, and if the problem is not addressed by the responsible managers, other colleagues can draw the conclusion that the organisation tolerates poor performance, and perhaps they too will work less or less well.

If the informal stage of managing the poorly performing colleague is not successful in leading to improvements, the manager will need to move to the **formal stage**.

We will not go into this in detail in this chapter because the formal stage is rather different in different organisations and contexts. Our impression, however, is that the manager needs to be even more familiar at the formal stage with the details of the organisation's policies, and to be quite sure to follow the procedures precisely so that the underperforming colleague is not able to claim that they have been unfairly treated. If possible, identify a specific person in your organisation's human resources department with whom you can liaise about the colleague concerned. There are likely to be **different pathways according to whether the question is of capability or conduct**. Being thorough in your role as the manager can also be stressful for you, especially if the situation may head towards a warning, sanction or dismissal for the employee. If you can, use your own supervision for support. Try to spend time with friends and colleagues to relax, although for reasons of confidentiality you will not be able to discuss with them the details of the poorly performing person. Although managing such situations can be difficult and sometimes conflictual, try to keep in mind the **'golden rule'**, namely, to treat the person you are managing as you would like to be treated, if your roles were reversed.

Key Points

- If you are trying to assist a colleague or peer who is performing poorly, decide clearly on what your role is and listen to what they have to say about their situation
- In particular, decide if you are able to discuss the person's issues in complete confidence or not
- If you are the manager of the poorly performing person, before addressing their performance become very familiar with the processes of your organisation, both to support the person and to manage that person's performance
- Manage poor performance through the informal and formal steps of your organisation

CHAPTER 25

How to Work in a Small Group

Work can be done on one's own or in a group. Working in a large group can assume the character of working in a small group – with a small number of members of the large group – or become similar to the work done on one's own. Working on one's own has the advantages of the freedom to decide how to organise one's day, and how and in what order to tackle priorities. It has the disadvantages that decisions have often to be taken without the **advice of others** with experience, that advice and **guidance by those with more experience** is not forthcoming, and that failures are much more difficult to overcome. Several other chapters are related to this topic.

Working with a group avoids some of the problems arising when working alone. The group often has members who have **experience of previous work on the same or similar tasks**. When decisions are difficult, the group can **discuss possible solutions** and make correct judgements with a good assessment of their advantages and disadvantages. Groups often have **formal or informal leaders** who can help in decision making and in finding solutions to problems. The group, if showing good cohesion, can **overcome periods of lesser energy** of its members, and often finds it possible to discover **solutions that none of its members working alone could find**.

A group that works well **produces more than the simple sum of achievements** of its members. Ill-functioning groups, however, produce significantly less than would be the sum of the individual products of members.

To be a good member of a group and to benefit from it requires several decisions by the individual who will join the group. Members of the group must **accept sharing the benefits** of their work. The way in which the benefits will be shared must be **settled in advance** by group consensus. An individual joining a group should raise the question of benefits and raise it when all the group members are present. The same is true for the division of work: if possible, the **decision about the distribution of work and responsibility** should be decided in a meeting of the group.

These suggestions are essential if the group creates itself by bringing together several people who would like to work together. The situation is somewhat different when an individual is invited or wishes to join a group that is already functioning. In such instances, the **newcomer will have to discuss the rights and responsibilities** with the leader of the group. Once this is done, it is helpful that the **leader announces the tasks and rights of the new member** in a meeting of the group. The announcement should be **detailed and clear**, rather than vague and short.

Once a member of a group, the newcomer should **invest time and effort to learn who the other members** of the group are, what they do, what they know, what they like and what they dislike. In medium-sized groups there are often factions: the new member of the group should learn about them, and try to act and be seen as a **friend of all members**. It is natural that friendship and closeness with other members of the group will differ from one to another member of the group. Not being a member of a faction or subgroup of a small group may have disadvantages, but which are usually less important than the gains from having friendly relations with all.

The interest in other members of the group should be permanent. It will require some time and effort to be up to date with the situation, wishes, disappointments and achievements of others but it is essential to do this. Friendships and **good relations with others are like flowers** – unless given time and water, flowers are likely to perish, and so it is also with friendship and good relations.

The new members of the group must try to learn as much as possible about other members and they should gain that knowledge by **disclosing information about themselves** and their preferences, hobbies, hopes and achievements (without bragging, letting the others discover the new member's assets). The new member should also **avoid critical comments** about the preferences of others and gossip about any subject or person. A general rule useful to remember is that one should try to learn as much as possible about the members of the group and **avoid confrontation** with any of them. If this is impossible, it is essential to search for another group that might be more congenial and harmonious with one's preferences, values and potentials.

Key Points

- Gain from the advice of more experienced members of the group
- Work together on possible solutions to difficult challenges
- Have clear allocations of roles and responsibilities
- New members should invest time to get to know other group members in detail
- Aim to establish and maintain positive working relationships with all group members
- Get to know other group members by disclosing information about yourself
- Avoid criticising or confronting other group members

CHAPTER 26

How to Reduce Tension in a Small Group or in a Meeting

Tensions in small groups are of two kinds: they can be **acute or longer lasting** (with or without an identifiable reason) or chronic. Lasting tensions make working in the group difficult and likely to contribute to a risk of burn-out of the group members. Sudden, unexpected tensions can become chronic unless they are dealt with without delay. This chapter is also related to several others, as shown below.

Acute Tension

The acute, unexpected tensions in a group are usually the result of one of three developments:

- the (often unexpected) **disclosure of information** about an event, a member of the group or another person linked in an important way to the work of the group
- a **change of the environment** of the group, influencing its action
- the unexpected and often **inexplicable behaviour** of one or more members of the group

Regardless of the reason for the sudden tension, the **leader of the group should interrupt the action in** which the group is engaged and either talk with the person causing the tension or explore the reasons for the change of environment that caused the tension.

The reaction to unexpected tension that occurs in a meeting should be handled by an interruption of the meeting and a **conversation with the person** who is at the origin of the tension. The discussion with the person who is at the core of the group's tension should take place in the same room in which the group is working, or nearby, in a place visible to all. If it appears that the discussion will take some considerable time, the leader of the group may have to stop the group work for an hour or two.

If the exploration will take even longer, the leader may need to dismiss the group until the reason for the tension has been clearly identified and dealt with.

Depending on the composition of the group, it might be necessary for the **conversation with the person at the centre of the problem to be carried out by a close friend or confidant** of the person whose disclosure, behaviour or statements caused the tension.

Often it is the manner of speaking rather than the content of what has been said that causes offence. If this is the case, it might take some time to change the behaviour of the person who has been the cause of tension. In some instances, it **might not be possible that such a person remains a member of the group** in which their behaviour is the reason for tension.

Sometimes the behaviour or the statements of the person who seems to be the cause of the tension is tolerable, even if not desirable, so this behaviour may not be sufficient to move the person to another group or work setting. This might be a situation in which the behaviour of a member of the group is for personal or other reasons, and may be unacceptable to only one or two members of the whole working group.

It might also be that a person's action or statements are considered unacceptable by one or two members of the group and that this is the consequence of **strongly held views** about a matter that has little or nothing to do with the tasks of the group. Thus a person who has strong views about the position of women or about the behaviour of men in their presence may resent the behaviour or statements of someone who does not fully share their views. In such situations it will be necessary that the leader speaks separately to both parties, trying to help them to **understand the other's position**, and to adjust their own behaviour to a level that will make collaboration possible.

Tension might also arise when the task of the team requires an **intensive investment of all members of the team** to make progress. To avoid tension and accusations that some of the team members "do not pull their weight", the team leader will have to spend time with each of the team members to ensure that they do not harbour ill feelings towards others, and to encourage each of the team members to do their best for the goals of the team.

The team leader has to spend their time in **constant contact** with the team members to discover dissatisfaction and tension early, as it is better dealt with before problems escalate. The time that the team leader spends in personal contact with each of the team members must be proportional to the amount of work that needs to be done.

It is particularly important to **be supportive to those who do best** – they are often investing themselves completely in the tasks at hand, which may lead to excessive fatigue and other consequences of working over one's limit.

The team leaders' time will have to be invested in the team's work and satisfaction in proportion to the amount of work that needs to be done. This means that **active support for feelings of achievement** and help to avoid a sense of incompetence resulting from minor failures and the other duties of leaders must be intensified, to make the team better achieve its objectives.

Longer-Term Tension

Lasting tensions might occur if the group has to work in a new setting that is unknown to some or all members of the group, making them feel less able to fulfil their duties. Lasting tensions can also be the result of the **failure to deal with acute tensions** at an earlier stage.

Most often, however, lasting tensions are found in teams whose members feel that no-one is **recognising and rewarding them for the value of the work** that the team is doing. The recognition of value is often late to come – after years of work it is recognised that a team has done marvellously well, but by that time the team members have often left, and others have joined. Those who have left feel that they should have been recognised for their work sooner, and the actual team members often do not feel that the recognition of the work that the team has done is sufficiently clearly and fully given to them.

Failure to achieve team goals is painful, particularly if the team members are committed to those goals. If nonachievement – regardless of its cause – becomes chronic, the team members will be embittered and often perform poorly or without joy. The role of the leaders is to ensure that the **achievements of the members of the team are well known, recognised and celebrated** by the team members themselves and by those around them.

The team leaders have to make sure that they remain aware and thankful for the achievement of the members of their team. They should also think of ways to follow the advice of team members about improvement and recognise publicly the improvements that have been achieved thanks to the suggestions of the team members, with **credit given where credit is due**.

Other reasons for the failure of teams and constant tensions are **team members who are not performing well** – either because they cannot do so or because they are not motivated to fully use their capacity. In relation to the first group, it will be a special duty of the team leaders to find tasks that members can do well and praise them for doing them well. For the second group, i.e., those who could do well if only they tried, the team leaders' task will be to increase their motivation, make them pull their weight, or remove them if efforts to motivate them and make them perform have not been successful. It is vital in both cases that the team leader actively addresses such problems of underperformance. It can be **highly corrosive to a team's ethos and motivation** if hardworking members see that less active team members can work less or less effectively with impunity and without any correction.

Tension in Meetings

Conducting meetings has much in common with leading teams. Meetings are much shorter and therefore it is necessary to act faster and avoid long-lasting plans about making meetings a success. The role of a smile or praise for a particularly useful suggestion becomes even more important than in the case of leading teams over a longer period of time. The time for exploring the feelings of the participants in a meeting is usually limited to the break times – or, in meetings that will last several days, to the evening hours and breakfast time. **Praise by the team leader** for particularly useful suggestions from team members must be given immediately, and preferably repeated.

Contact with those participating in a meeting requires **constant attention to body language** – seeing which proposals are met with signs of rejection or incredulity; seeing which of the participants avoid looking at the speaker with whom they do not agree. Signs of boredom in the meeting participants should be taken seriously and corrected by an apposite remark, a witty comment, or a parable bringing the wider background of the boring part into connection by using relevant topics.

The chairperson of the meeting must, among other preparations for the meeting, spend time thinking about the participants, their previous work and their individual interests. It is the role of the **chairperson to bring out the best in the participants** and make them play roles in which they are excellent. Thus, for example, someone who is good at making summaries should be invited to do so in the course of the meeting, and others who are particularly familiar with the background literature should be invited to produce relevant references, and so on, to play to their strengths.

The chairperson, as the leader of a group, should try to **identify the strength of links between those present in the meeting** – as group leaders would explore the strength of friendships among the members of the team – and gain insight into the strength of authority that members of the group, and the participants in a meeting, are likely to have.

In trying to reduce tensions in a small group or in a meeting, it can be **dangerous to use humorous** remarks to resolve problems. Although the tension might become less strong or visible after all have laughed, the basic problems that have led to tension remain unresolved by laughter alone. Even making jokes about oneself or one's own weakness is not useful: the laughter will take away the bitterness, but it may do so before the problems are resolved, which hides them instead of resolving them.

Key Points

- The team leader needs to identify the cause of tensions within a work group
- If tensions arise in a group meeting, it may be necessary to stop the meeting and directly address the person who seems to be the source of the tension
- Where there are deep-seated reasons for behaviour by a team member that is not acceptable to others, this person may need to leave the group or team
- It is necessary for team leaders to address sources of tension or friction in a group or team
- The leader will usually want to try to help team members who are in conflict, to understand the point of view of others
- Efforts by the team leader should be proportionate to the scale of the tension or problem, with much effort retained to praise staff who are doing well, recognising and rewarding their work
- Identify the strengths of each team leader and encourage them to contribute these skills to the objectives of the team

CHAPTER 27

How to Be a Mentor Or a Mentee

This chapter outlines a particular approach to mentoring, with our views on how to make the best of such a relationship from the perspectives of the mentor and the mentee. We also include practical materials to support mentorship.

What Is Mentorship?

Most writers agree that mentoring is a relationship between a more senior (mentor) and a less senior colleague (mentee), designed to guide, help and support the latter. It is not a directive activity – the mentor does not tell the mentee what to do. It is important to emphasise that the mentor role is distinct from the supervisor role, so that the mentor must not have any formal line management responsibility for the mentee, and indeed the two may be employed by different organisations.

Mentees are responsible for setting their own goals and overall development, and the mentor's role is to listen and advise the mentee where appropriate, to ensure the mentee develops professionally to their full capability. A constructive relationship between the mentor and mentee is essential to achieving a successful mentoring outcome. A high degree of mutual trust between the mentor and mentee is needed to realise the full potential of a mentorship relationship.

Mentoring is **distinct from other supportive relationships**, such as coaching, counselling or supervision. Our colleagues Dr Petra Gronholm and Professor Heidi Lempp at King's College, London, have described mentoring as an effective way to provide encouragement, support and motivation to someone, and we are pleased to acknowledge their contributions towards the ideas included in this chapter (Gronholm et al., 2023). Table 27.1 outlines how these types of engagement differ from one another.

Why Be a Mentor?

The role of mentor is usually held by a person within an organisation who has a relatively **high level of experience or seniority**. Such people often have multiple and complex responsibilities, so why take on the role of mentor? Many senior staff feel a need to **leave a legacy** from their work that will be sustained in the future – to contribute to the continuation of their vocation through passing on their knowledge and wisdom to others, both people within their own organisation and people

TABLE 27.1 ■ Overview of Differences Between Mentoring, Coaching, Counselling and Supervision

	Mentoring	Coaching	Counselling	Supervision
Focus	Present and future	Present and future	Past and its impact on the present	Present and future
Key goal	To support personal and professional development	To correct or optimise behaviours to improve performance, and impart skills	Resolve psychosocial issues, support personal wellbeing	To monitor performance in relation to specific work-related responsibilities
Agenda	Set by mentee with mentor providing support, guidance, and experience sharing	Set by individuals with coach assisting in achieving specific goals	Set by individuals and counsellors aimed at achieving short-term or long-term goals	Set by supervisor/ manager (or higher management)
Engagement period	Ongoing relationship that can last for a long period	Relationship is for a short duration	Relationship is short-term but can last longer due to breadth of issues being addressed	Duration of employment contract
Training	Experience and training	Often accredited	Certified health professional	Professional experience; might include specific training
Learning	Two-way (mentoring interaction can be rewarding and lead to new insights for both mentors and mentees)	One-way (the person being mentored is the main beneficiary)	One-way (the person receiving counselling is the main beneficiary)	One-way (the employee is accountable to the supervisor/manager)

working elsewhere. It is usual that the mentor is a more senior or a more experienced individual than the mentee.

Preparing to Be a Mentor

Mentor–mentee dyads can be formed on an ad hoc basis, or in a purposive and structured way. This chapter outlines a rather **structured approach to setting up mentorship,** but many of the characteristics of successful mentorship outlined here will work equally well if the relationship is set up individually, either initiated by the mentor or by the mentee.

Steps in Mentorship

We base this chapter upon the mentorship approach developed for the Indigo Partnership Programme. This was a research programme funded by the UK Medical Research Council to develop effective interventions to reduce mental health-related stigma in China, Ethiopia, India, Nepal and Tunisia (Gronholm et al., 2023). The scheme aimed to support early career researchers (ECR) in these countries by pairing ECRs with more senior colleagues within the Indigo programme, following the stepwise process shown in Appendix 27.5.

Mentorship Scheme Objectives

A mentorship scheme may have a series of **preset objectives,** for example:
- To match ECR mentees with a career mentor whose background and skills are compatible with the mentee's career aspirations.
- To develop a mentoring relationship that fosters supportive, encouraging and goal-orientated discussions.
- To provide regular opportunities to explore ECR mentees' short- and long-term career development goals.
- To identify opportunities to support these career development goals through activities related to the ECR mentee's role.
- To provide a safe space for ECR mentees to explore barriers to skill and career development and to be supported to identify their own solutions.

Commitment Required to a Mentorship Scheme

We suggest a somewhat structured approach to mentorship so that the **expectations for the mentor and the mentee are reasonably clear and aligned** from the outset, including, for example:
- Mentees and mentors to familiarise themselves with a Mentoring Scheme Handbook and other practical materials before starting the programme.
- To jointly complete a Mentoring Agreement.
- To arrange to meet on a regular basis.

- Mentees to prepare for meetings and work towards identified career development goals.
- To provide constructive and meaningful feedback for evaluation purposes.
- To contact the scheme coordinators in a timely manner if there are any concerns.
- A mentorship relationship may be for a specific time period, or may continue for longer, indeed over many years.

Establishing the Baseline Before Starting Mentorship

As a starting point for the career development scheme, ECRs are encouraged to **reflect on their current career stage**, and how and where they would like to progress next.

ECRs should **identify short-, medium- and long-term goals** that could help them to progress their career. These goals will form the basis of the initial meeting with the mentor.

Initial Goal-Setting Meeting

The next step in the career development **mentoring process** is the first meeting between the mentor and mentee. This meeting is an opportunity for both to have an initial discussion about the mentee's views about their career goals. The mentor can then review the career development goals presented by the mentee and work with them to identify a small number of objectives to achieve during the mentorship period, including actions to be completed before the next meeting.

During this meeting the mentee and mentor can also discuss how they would like to incorporate **recommended resources** such as the GROW model (see Appendix 27.1) into their discussions and utilise the SMART Goals framework (see Appendix 27.2) to work towards clear and agreed career development goals. Do keep in mind the distinct roles and responsibilities of the mentor and the mentee (see Appendix 27.3).

We suggest that you consider using a Mentoring Agreement form (see Appendix 27.4), outlining the **principles that have been jointly agreed** on for the mentoring relationship. Specifically, the pair can discuss and agree on when and how subsequent follow-up meetings will be scheduled; the boundaries of the mentoring relationship; rules about confidentiality, and when appropriate to signpost to other relevant sources of support; expectations about follow-up contact between meetings; and contact preferences for both the mentor and the mentee. This document is to be jointly completed and signed by each, so both have a written record of what they have agreed on for their mentoring relationship.

Mentorship Meeting Preparation

After the initial goal-setting meeting, follow-up meetings with the mentor are to be **scheduled on a regular basis**, for example, every 3 months, in addition to an annual meeting to review the previous year and to set goals for the next year. Arranging these meetings is expected to be *led by the mentee*. It is the mentee's responsibility to contact the mentor and arrange meetings, decide on the content (career development goals) to be discussed at the meetings, to prepare an agenda and other relevant materials ahead of the meetings (e.g., the completed SMART Goals template, and progress towards the goals) and to share these with the mentor ahead of the meeting, as per the procedures outlined in the Mentoring Agreement.

Follow-Up Meetings

During these meetings, the mentor and mentee review the career development goals that were set during their previous meeting and discuss progress towards reaching these goals. During the follow-up meeting new or updated goals can be decided for the next follow-up meeting.

Annual Goal-Review Meeting

At the beginning of each annual mentoring cycle, an **updated goal-setting meeting** can be arranged for the mentor and mentee. At this meeting, progress towards the goals set for the previous year is discussed, and a modified plan may need to be agreed to make progress towards the mentee's longer-term goals. During this meeting the mentor and mentee can review the Mentoring Agreement.

Ending a Mentoring Relationship

We suggest that a mentoring relationship is set up for a fixed-term period, for example for 1, 2 or 3 years. This gives a clear shape to the time available to make progress towards the mentee's goals. At the end of this period, both may agree to extend the relationship, and again we suggest that this is for a defined period. If the relationship proves to be mutually rewarding, such mentorship may continue fruitfully over many years, across periods of career transitions for both mentor and mentee.

Further Information

These sources may offer additional helpful material on mentoring:
   https://www.mindtools.com/pages/article/newLDR_89.htm
   http://www.studylecturenotes.com/management/john-whitmore-grow-model-a-coaching-mentoring-process
   https://www.performanceconsultants.com/grow-model
   https://www.mindtools.com/pages/article/smart-goals.htm
   https://www.smartsheet.com/blog/essential-guide-writing-smart-goals

Appendix 27.1 The GROW Model

The GROW model is a four-step process that can be used for structuring the mentoring processes and to reflect on how to explore directions and priorities for career development (Fig. 27.1).

The GROW model is useful to help a person identify their priorities and improve their performance, to facilitate planning and reaching career objectives. It provides a useful tool to highlight, elicit and maximise potential through a series of sequential coaching conversations.

The implementation of the GROW model can be conceptualised as planning a career journey. You need to decide where you will go (the *Goal*), and where your current location is (your *Reality*, the current situation). You also need to think about the various ways and means (the *Options*) to reach on your decided location, and ultimately work out a plan for your travels and make the necessary preparations, committing to following through the plan of action you have decided on (the *Will*).

By working through these four stages, the GROW model raises the mentee's awareness and understanding of:

- their own aspirations
- their current situation and beliefs
- the possibilities and resources open to them
- the actions they want to take to achieve their personal and professional goals

HOW TO USE THE GROW MODEL

The following steps are involved in a mentoring process structured by the GROW model.

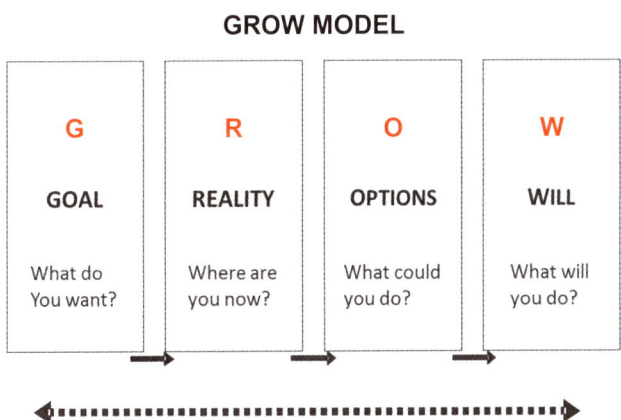

Fig. 27.1   The GROW model

1 ESTABLISH THE *GOAL*

In the first step of the model you need to define the *Goal*. This can involve thinking about the professional and/or academic behaviour or situation that you want to change. This desired change will be the goal you want to achieve.

At this stage it is useful to consider the following:

- How will you know that the goal is achieved? How will you know that the problem or issue is solved?
- Does the goal fit with the mentee's overall career objectives? Does it fit with the team's objectives?

By setting goals that are relevant and challenging, as well as specific, measurable and achievable, in a realistic time frame, the GROW model can promote confidence and self-motivation, leading to increased productivity and personal satisfaction. It is useful to define the goal in terms of the SMART Goals framework, i.e., to ensure the goal is Specific, Measurable, Attainable, Realistic, and Time-bound. This framework is explained in more detail in the next section.

2 EXAMINE THE CURRENT *REALITY*

In this step of the GROW model you need to consider the current *Reality* (position) of the person wishing to action change.

This is an important step but usually people try to reach a goal or solve a problem without fully considering their starting point. Without clearly examining the current reality that a person is experiencing, there is a possible risk of missing some information that could be required to achieve the defined goal effectively.

At this stage it is useful to consider the following:

- What is the current situation, and what is happening towards achieving the goal?
- Does the current reality already reflect steps taken towards reaching the defined goal?
- Does the defined goal conflict with any other goals and objectives?

3 EXPLORE THE *OPTIONS*

Once the current reality is recognised, the mentor/mentee can determine what is possible. In this step it is important to explore as many *Options* as possible for achieving defined goals and objectives.

At this stage, it might be useful to brainstorm different ideas. When a range of options is identified, these solutions can be discussed and the best one(s) selected.

Mentees and mentors might have different perspectives regarding different options. It is important to collaboratively agree on what the most effective and appropriate options might be, as this develops a sense of ownership and agency that can help keep up motivation for achieving the defined goals and objectives.

At this stage it is useful to consider the following:

- What else could you do?
- What if this or that constraint was removed? Would that change things?
- What are the advantages and disadvantages of each option?
- What factors or considerations will you use to weigh the options?
- What do you need to stop doing to achieve this goal?
- What obstacles stand in your way?

4 AGREED ACTIONS

The *Will* element of the model is the barometer of success. It relates to aspiration, desire and intention. By examining the current reality and exploring the options, it is easier to see how a given goal can be achieved. The final important step is to commit to specific actions to move forward towards practically attain the defined goal.

At this stage it is useful to consider the following:

- What will you do now, how will you move forward?
- What else will you do to proceed better?
- What could stop you moving forward? How will you overcome this?
- How can you keep yourself committed and motivated?
- On which basis will you need to review progress? And how often – daily, weekly, monthly?

Appendix 27.2 SMART Goals

SMART Goals is a tool to guide your goal-setting by providing a framework within which to create criteria to help improve the chances of succeeding in accomplishing a goal.

This framework is intended to help you develop clear and reachable goals, through formulating goals in a way that make them **S**pecific, **M**easurable, **A**chievable, **R**elevant, and **T**ime-bound. The SMART Goals template below can be used to structure goals in line with these SMART principles.

SMART GOALS TEMPLATE

Initial goal. Write the goal you have in mind.
Specific. What exactly do you want to accomplish? Who needs to be included? When do you want to do this? Why is this a goal?
Measurable. How can you measure progress and know if you have successfully met your goal?
Achievable. Do you have the skills required to achieve the goal? If not, can you obtain them? What is the motivation for this goal? Is the amount of effort required on par with what the goal will achieve?
Relevant. Why am I setting this goal now? Is it aligned with overall objectives?

Time-bound. What is the deadline and is it realistic?

SMART Goal: Review your initial goal statement in view of your answers to the questions above, and revise the goal as appropriate to align it with the SMART framework principles.

SMART Goals Principles Explained

Goal-setting can be refined through considering the goals in terms of the following five aspects of the SMART framework:

1 SPECIFIC

What exactly is it that you want to achieve?

Your goals need be clear and specific, otherwise you will not be able to focus your efforts or stay motivated to achieve them. When you draft your goal, try to answer the 'five Ws' questions:

- **Who** is involved? Who needs to be involved (this is especially important when you are working on a group project)?
- **What** do I want to accomplish? Exactly what are you trying to accomplish? Do not be afraid to get very detailed.
- **Where** is it located? This question may not always apply, especially if you are setting personal goals, but if there is a location or relevant event, identify it here.
- **Which** resources or limits are involved? Determine any related obstacles or requirements. This question can be beneficial in deciding if your goal is realistic.
- **Why** is this goal important? What is the reason for the goal? Why does it matter?

2 MEASURABLE

How will you know that you have achieved the goal?

It is important to have measurable goals, so that you can track your progress and stay motivated. Assessing progress helps you to stay focused, meet your deadlines, and feel the excitement of getting closer to achieving your goal.

A measurable goal may address the following questions:
- How much?
- How many?
- How will I know when it is accomplished?

3 ACHIEVABLE

Is the goal feasible within the time frame?

Your goal also needs to be realistic and attainable to be successful. In other words, it needs to stretch your abilities but still remain possible. The goal is meant to inspire motivation, not discouragement. When you set an achievable goal, you may be able to identify previously overlooked opportunities or resources that can bring you closer to it. If you set your target too high it can cause stress and decrease the chance of reaching your target, which can lead to demotivation.

Think about how to accomplish the goal and if you have the tools/skills needed. If you do not currently possess those tools/skills, consider what it would take to attain them.

An achievable goal will usually answer questions such as:
- How can I accomplish this goal?
- How realistic is the goal, based on other constraints such as time or financial factors?

4 RELEVANT

Does this goal contribute towards your long-term plans, and does it fit within the research team's plans?

This step is about ensuring that your goal matters to you, and, if relevant, that it also aligns with other relevant goals the person or team is pursuing. We all need support and assistance in achieving our goals, but it is important to retain control over them. So, make sure that your plans drive everyone forward, but that you are still responsible for achieving your own goal.

A relevant goal can answer 'yes' to these questions:
- Does this seem worthwhile?
- Is this the right time?
- Does this match our other efforts/needs?
- Am I the right person to reach this goal?
- Is it applicable in the current socioeconomic environment?

5 TIME-BOUND

By what date will this objective be achieved?

Every goal needs a target date, so that you have a deadline to focus on and something to work towards. This part of the SMART Goal criteria helps to prevent everyday tasks from taking priority over your longer-term goals.

Anyone can set goals, but if they lack realistic timing, chances are you are not going to reach them. Providing a target date for deliverables is imperative. Ask specific questions about the goal deadline and what can be accomplished within that time period. If the goal will take 3 months to complete, it is useful to define what should be achieved halfway through the process. Providing time constraints also creates a sense of urgency.

A time-bound goal will usually answer these questions:

- When?
- What can I do 6months from now?
- What can I do 6 weeks from now?
- What can I do today?

Appendix 27.3 Roles of Mentor/Mentee

THE ROLES OF THE MENTOR

Helps the mentee to clarify thoughts and goals, and to find their own solutions

Encourages the mentee to drive the partnership

Helps the mentee deal with both short-term problems and long-term development

Supports, listens and constructively challenges the mentee

THE ROLES OF THE MENTEE

Drives partnership, initiating regular contact

Sets realistic expectations

Sets and works towards SMART Goals

Listens, is open to and responds to constructive feedback by the mentor

Seeks own solutions to challenges

Engages in their own learning and development

Works on goals between sessions

WAYS IN WHICH MENTORS CAN SUPPORT MENTEES

Improving personal effectiveness (e.g., organisational skills, time management, workload management, setting achievable goals)

Leadership skills, management roles

Promotion, career progression (e.g., identifying options, interview skills, preparing for appraisals)

Strengthening scientific communication (e.g., publications, presentation and public speaking skills)

Reviewing transferrable skills

Applying for grant funding

Teaching

Growing professional networks, building networking skills

Building links with stakeholders, public engagement, other outreach

Planning for/returning back from a career break or other longer period of leave

Working part-time or flexible hours; work/life balance

Handling challenging situations (e.g., conflict in the workplace, overcoming barriers to progression, managing cultural differences and/or expectations, managing working relationships)

WHAT THE MENTOR IS NOT

A mentor will not solve the mentee's problems, or offer magical solutions

A mentor may have less time than the mentee

The mentor is not expected to open doors (provide job opportunities, etc.)

The mentor may be prepared to share their experiences, but remember that everybody's circumstances are different

A mentor may not be around forever

Appendix 27.4 Mentoring Agreement Form

DRAFT MENTORING AGREEMENT

To be discussed and signed by both the mentor and mentee

We agree to:
- Meet, speak or email on a regular basis.
- Provide feedback and evaluation as requested.
- Review our progress regularly against our objectives/plan.
- Respect the development aims of the Indigo Partnership ECR mentoring programme
- If we cannot attend a scheduled meeting/telephone conversation, we agree to notify our partner and reschedule well in advance if possible.
- We agree that if for any reason either of us is not comfortable in our mentoring relationship, we can end the mentoring contact after consulting with the mentoring scheme coordinators.

We will arrange to meet regularly and have discussed how these meetings will be arranged. Our plan is to:	
We will discuss the boundaries of the mentoring relationship and agree on some objectives and broad topic areas we will explore during the mentoring. These are:	
We will abide by the confidentiality rules we choose. These are:	
We agree to jointly identify other sources of support to contact for areas that are beyond what is appropriate to consider within a mentoring context. This might involve, for example:	
We will discuss the level of follow-up contact and actions (if any) we expect/prefer between meetings. This is:	
We will discuss contact preferences. The best way/time to reach us is:	
Mentor:	
Mentee:	
Mentor Signature	Mentee Signature
Date	Date

Appendix 27.5 Steps of a Mentorship Programme

Establishing the baseline

• ECR mentee reflects on current career stage, and identifies potential career development goals (short-term, medium-term, and long-term).

Initial annual goal-setting meeting

• ECR mentee schedules first meeting with mentor, during which thoughts around career development and potential career development goals are discussed.

• Mentor introduces GROW model and SMART framework

• The ECR mentee and mentor decide on longer-term goals to focus on in the coming year, and 2-3 short-term goals for working towards the long-term goal during the next quarter.

• Mentoring Agreement form to be completed.

Meeting preparation

• ECR mentee formulates longer-term and short-term goals within the SMART framework, and schedules a follow-up meeting with the mentor to discuss career development goals and progress.

• *Follow-up meetings are to be scheduled quarterly; i.e., three follow-up meetings per year, in addition to the annual goal-setting meeting.*

Follow-up meetings

• Scheduling of and preparing for meeting to be led by the mentee.

• ECR mentee and mentor discuss progress towards the previously identified goals, and decide on new/updated goals for the next follow-up meeting.

Annual goal-setting meeting

• At the end of the year the ECR arranges another joint meeting with the mentor, during which progress towards the past year's goals is discussed.

• The mentee and mentor decide on new longer-term goal for next year, and 2-3 short-term goals for working towards longer-term goal during the next quarter.

• Mentoring Agreement form to be reviewed.

Fig. 27.5 Indigo Partnership ECR career development scheme. From: Gronholm PC, Bakolis I, Cherian AV, et al. Toward a multi-level strategy to reduce stigma in global mental health: overview protocolcof the Indigo Partnership to develop and test interventions in low- and middle-income countries. *Int J Ment Health Syst* 2023; 17(1): 2.

CHAPTER 28

How to Collaborate, and Use Networks and Feedback

Knowing how to work well with colleagues is an essential set of skills for most student and qualified professionals. To a very great extent these are learnable skills. In this chapter we focus on three specific aspects of team and group working: how to collaborate, how to use networks and how to give and receive feedback. Many of the other chapters in this book discuss other important aspects of collaborative working styles and methods, as shown in the box below.

RELATED CHAPTERS

Chapter 8. How to work with people from other cultures
Chapter 14. How to take part in a meeting
Chapter 16. How to lead a small working group or collaboration
Chapter 19. How to take part in a video meeting
Chapter 22. How to negotiate
Chapter 25. How to work in a small group
Chapter 27. How to be a mentor or a mentee
Chapter 31. How to work well in video and online collaborations

How to Collaborate

We *defined a collaboration* in Chapter 16 (concerned with leading consortia) as '*a group of participants who have a common purpose and who have complementary skills, and between whom all the necessary types of expertise are included in the group*'. A primary consideration in participating in any specific collaboration, rather than leading it, is to *know clearly what the purpose of the collaboration is*.

Once the purpose has been clarified, an important series of further questions arise about how the collaboration will start, continue and complete its work.

ESSENTIAL QUESTIONS TO ADDRESS IN SETTING UP A COLLABORATION

- Who is in the group?
- What are the roles of each participant?

- What is each person expected to do, and when, with whom and with what resources?
- Do any individuals or groups need *training or support* to fully play their parts?
- Exactly what is expected to be achieved or delivered by each person, each team and by the collaboration as a whole?
- *Who is coordinating* the whole consortium?
- How do they *know what is happening* across the programme?
- Who has *authority to allocate resources* for each component of the whole programme, and to hold members of the group to account if work is not done as agreed?
- Where tasks have been allocated to different members of the whole group or to subgroups, has this been by mutual agreement?
- Have intermediate and final *deadlines* for deliverables been *negotiated or imposed?*
- To whom does progress need to be reported and in what degree of detail and in what format?

Participants in any collaboration are very unlikely to be entirely altruistic. There is usually a balance to be struck between *what group members give and what they expect to take* from the collaboration. Another way to consider this is to try to understand the *needs of all other group members* and to see, as far as possible, how these needs can be met while also achieving the purpose of the collaboration.

Collaborations usually succeed faster and more easily if there is at least a reasonable *level of trust* between group members. At least in the early stages of any consortium, we strongly suggest that group members arrange to *meet in person* to begin to get to know and to trust each other. If this foundation is laid well in the early stage of a programme, then video or remote contact at a later stage may be sufficient for regular communication, but with some periodic in-person meetings to give a booster to the human side of the equation.

Whatever the nature of the collaboration, it will be helpful to identify at the outset hotspots or *probable flash points* that could present a risk to the viability of the programme, and that specific methods to mitigate these risks are taken. For example, for in-service development projects, we suggest that the *budget allocation* is very clear to all senior participants. For academic collaborations we suggest a clear formal written agreement is drawn up on how the *authorship of scientific papers* will be managed, and that this is completed within the first few months of the collaboration.

Also identify at an early stage in the collaborative programme, or even before the start if a detailed proposal has been written, for example, to gain funding, exactly *how conflicts will be managed* and what stages will be used for *conflict resolution*. While hoping that this will not be necessary, disputes between team members or partners can arise, and in that case the group will not want to spend time inventing a method to deal with this – the procedure can be agreed in advance. If you are involved in a disagreement or conflict within the work group, first of all see if you can *resolve this informally*, and start by doing your best to understand the *other person's point of view*.

Expect that some people in a collaboration will *change over time*, including key members. If you can, build *flexibility or resilience* into the structure of the collaboration, for example, by having deputies to lead roles, or by having two leads for important programme components. Many programmes face challenges along the way, typically slowing down at the midway point. We suggest that you develop in your collaborations not only ways to identify problems, such as overdue or incomplete tasks, but that you also take every opportunity to *celebrate success* among your team members. No success is too small to be suitable for congratulation.

To help manage a large-scale programme, we suggest you have an *ongoing framework of regular meetings*, to give a clear structure and rhythm for discussing the work of the group, and to prevent usually the need to have crisis meetings. Encourage a culture in your team of *sharing challenges when they appear early on*, while they are still small enough to be relatively easily to remedy.

How to Use Networks

We see networking as a way to create a woven fabric of personal contacts, who can give you *time, understanding, challenge, feedback, support, insight, formal and informal information, and resources*. Often this will be on a peer support or mutual self-help basis. Where there is an asymmetry in the direction of assistance, this can more closely resemble mentoring (see Chapter 27).

We suggest that you look upon networking as a *long-term part of your career plans*. Among the many people you come across in your work, in your own organisation, or in other countries, there will be some for whom you feel a particular affinity, liking or respect. We suggest that *mutual regard and respect* is a sound starting point for new members of your network, not simply a utilitarian view of who you can use in the future. Keep in mind that both for the closer and the more distant members of your network, you will not know when you will need to call on them for assistance until an event, or even a crisis, occurs in your life, for example, suddenly finding yourself facing unemployment.

Your network needs to be both *created and maintained*. Starting a potentially long-term and positive work-related meeting is best done, in our view, in person. This could be with a short discussion before or after a work meeting, or at a social event, or when you deliberately contact a person and arrange to meet because you have a shared interest. Bear in mind that network members will usually offer a *reciprocal advantage*. What is it you can offer to your colleague and what can they offer you. Is this a balanced, nonexploitative equation? Have a *paper or electronic personal card* ready when you meet new people at work events, and be ready to offer this to people who you find interesting in your field. Immediately after the first meeting, follow up with a short and positive note to say how much you enjoyed meeting the person and how you hope that you can both stay in touch.

Maintaining contact with a person in your network is also vital. One approach is to act a *'little and often'*. If you notice a relevant news story or recent publication you can send this or a weblink to the person saying that this might be of interest.

If you are going to a congress, you can send a short note to ask if they are going and suggest you meet up for a coffee. Be prepared to initiate contacts, as the other person may not have remembered you clearly from a first meeting or may not be so active in maintaining their own network. Be *relentlessly positive* in your series of contacts with the other person. If you need assistance with a particular work-related challenge you have, be ready to *send out an inquiry* to some or all of your network. Be aware that members of your network may not know each other, and you do not necessarily have their permission to share their details with others, so either write to people individually, or send a group letter while *protecting the anonymity* of colleagues by using the 'blind copy' facility of your email. By the same token, if members of your network write to you asking for help, try hard to assist them. As we saw in Chapter 11 on how to chair a meeting, contacts with colleagues in your network can be more rewarding and memorable if you combine technical/operational and relational/emotional types of communication in your meeting.

An interesting paper by Ibarra and Hunter in the Harvard Business Review has described *three different types of networking*: operational, personal and strategic, as shown in Table 28.1. As you build your network, you can observe which of these types is most helpful to you.

As you expand your network, you can consider *several stages* to this process. Establish your *core work-related identity*, for example, with a short form of your curriculum vitae (see Chapter 32), called a biography or 'brief bio'. You also want to create *your own website* or LinkedIn web presence. On these sites include links to the aspects of your work or achievements that you are most proud. This is called *setting up your portfolio*. Send these links to members of your network and ask them to pass the links on to colleagues of theirs who have similar interests. Make a *bridge between your online and offline worlds*. For example, if you are going to a national or international meeting, include this news on your website or social media page and say you would be happy to arrange an in-person meeting with members of your network. When you have a contact with a network member, and if you agree to carry out a task, *be sure to follow up* and to do this promptly. Not delivering or doing this slowly can weaken a network link. Being *sincere and trustworthy* will, in the long run, greatly enhance your personal reputation.

How to Use Feedback

By now you will have realised that we end many chapters in this book by encouraging you to *actively seek, consider and use feedback* from other people to help you to refine your leadership skills. The reason is that, in our view, many of these skills are ones that you can learn and then improve over time, and that such *learning is accelerated by using feedback*. In this section we focus on using feedback to you from other people, but you may find that many of these points will also assist you when you offer feedback to others.

In a technical or engineering sense, feedback can mean 'the communication of evaluative or corrective information about an action, event, or process to the original

TABLE 28.1 ■ **The Three Forms of Networking**

Managers Who Think They Are Adept At Networking Are Often Operating Only At An Operational Or Personal Level. Effective Leaders Learn To Employ Networks For Strategic Purposes.

	Operational	**Personal**	**Strategic**
Purpose	Getting work done efficiently: maintaining the capacities and functions required of the group.	Enhancing personal and professional development; providing referrals to useful information and contacts.	Figuring out future priorities and challenges; getting stakeholder support for them.
Location and temporal orientation	Contacts are mostly internal and orientated towards current demands.	Contacts are mostly external and orientated towards current interests and future potential interests.	Contacts are internal and external and orientated towards the future.
Players and recruitment	Key contacts are relatively nondiscretionary; they are prescribed mostly by the task and organisational structure, so it is very clear who is relevant.	Key contacts are mostly discretionary; it is not always clear who is relevant.	Key contacts follow from the strategic context and the organisational environment, but specific membership is discretionary; it is not always clear who is relevant.
Network attributes and key behaviours	Depth: building strong working relationships.	Breadth: reaching out to contacts who can make referrals.	Leverage: creating inside–outside links.

(From Ibarra and Hunter, 2017)

or controlling source' or the 'return to the input of a part of the output of a machine, system, or process'. Now let's transform this into what feedback means for a human process or system. In this chapter we use feedback to mean *'the purposive gathering, weighing, and use of information of one aspect of your work, designed to improve your performance of that task'*. For example, you had to give an oral presentation at a professional meeting. You felt very nervous and you do not know if it went well or badly. Arrange, preferably in advance of the meeting, for a few colleagues to assess how well you do and to give you their honest comments soon after the meeting. If it might help you or them, their comments can be anonymised. Explain that although you hope that some of their comments will be positive, their *most useful comments are more likely to indicate where and how you can improve* how you do that particular task, for example, comments on speaking more slowly or parts of your talk that were less engaging or even boring. You want usable information, not only about areas for improvement, but also *very specific suggestions* about what you can do better next time, that is, aspects of your work that you can change.

Look at the feedback a little later when your elation or despondency immediately after the meeting has subsided. Try to read the feedback you get as if it is not about you but about another person, that is, *depersonalise the comments*. By all means take some credit for what you did well. But if you receive any adverse comments, tell yourself that this is not about you as a person, but about your behaviour on that particular occasion. Usually people pay about three times more attention to the criticism than to the praise they receive – try to give a balance to both. Sometimes it will be helpful to seek *information on comparators*, for example, how well did you give your first presentation to this group of colleagues compared with others giving their first presentation?

We suggest that you form *peer groups* for different aspects of your work – groups that can regularly give feedback to one another, both during your professional training and after you have qualified in your chosen field. Such feedback can be *peer-directed* (to colleagues at your level), *upward* (to more senior colleagues), *downward* (to more junior colleagues) or *coaching* (helping the other person to identify a challenge, identify options, appraise these options, decide what to do, and then do it). Another type of feedback is given live. For example, in a role play for a trainee doctor with a patient, the session leader can use the '*stop–start*' technique to interrupt the role play and to invite comments from the two participants and from the group members. A variant of this is to *audio- or video-record*, for example, a clinical meeting between a junior nurse and a patient, after which the teacher replays the meeting with the clinician, or perhaps also with the patient, to check what they were thinking and feeling at key points of the meeting, and what other options the practitioner had at these turning points.

Ways to Actively Receive Feedback

- Pay careful attention (several times) to what is said or written about you
- Gracefully and briefly accept praise
- Try not to become defensive if some comments are negative
- Seek clarification if you do not understand any comment clearly
- Do not interrupt or argue with the person giving you feedback
- Focus on what is said to you and do not feel you have to quickly accept or reject it
- You may want to ask what you could have done differently
- Towards the end of the feedback session, thank the person for their time and trouble

A recent development is called *360-degree feedback*. This means that several people, for example, 10–20, are asked to give feedback about one member of staff, usually using an online system, and often anonymously. Responses are then summarised by the feedback system and the results are fed back to the person concerned. For example, a doctor may hear that 94% of his patients rated her as 'trustworthy in their clinical practice', and that the average rating for doctors in that hospital in that year was 92% for this question. This therefore offers helpful absolute and relative information for this doctor, sometimes displayed graphically, for example, using a spider chart, to assess how well they are doing on this issue.

Apart from feedback from peers, another option is *feedback by managers* to the people they manage. This can be feedback rated by the manager, or a synthesis of feedback information from other colleagues. In this case the feedback will often be discussed in the context of a regular *performance review or appraisal meeting*. The same principles given previously apply here. In addition, the manager is likely to summarise the key areas where tasks can be done better, to agree what actions the employee will take, and when this will be reviewed next.

A report by Hardavella and colleagues (2017) provides a practical summary of many issues related to feedback. The box below shows *who can provide feedback* in clinical settings, and in Fig. 28.1 they summarise important points to keep in mind about feedback.

Important Types of Feedback in the Health Care Professions (Hardavella et al., 2017)

- Informal feedback is the most frequent form and is provided on a day-to-day basis, by any member of the team.
- Formal feedback comes as part of a structured assessment, usually provided in writing by peers or superiors.
- Formative feedback is about a learner's progress at a particular time during a course of instruction or during the acquisition of a new skill, and it relies on continuous encouragement.
- Summative feedback measures performance, often against a standard, and comes with a mark or grade and feedback to explain your mark. It can be used to rank or judge individuals and to assess if they have reached the required standard of performance to qualify as a professional.

Source: Hardavella et al., 2017.

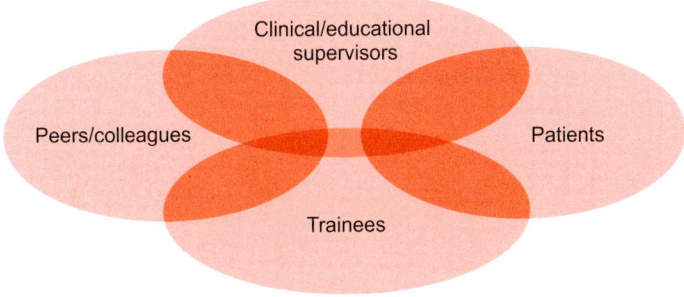

Fig. 28.1   Sources of feedback for clinical staff

Tips on Giving Effective Feedback

- Plan in advance.
- Give the feedback promptly, right after the event.
- Consider what you want to achieve and shape the meeting in this way.
- Feedback is usually better if provided directly to the person.
- Consider the 'sandwich': a positive comment, then a negative comment, then positive.
- Be specific about what you feel can be improved and also say how, with an example.
- Look for nonverbal indication from the other person of how they are receiving feedback.
- Ask the person to reflect on the task being assessed. What went well? What did not go well? Why not?
- Ask the person 'What would you do differently next time?' and 'What have you learned from this session?'

Key Points

Collaboration

- Identify clearly the purpose of the collaboration
- Be clear about your role in the collaboration and the roles of others
- Meet in person early in the programme to start to establish trust
- Include technical and relational aspects into your meetings
- Identify in advance probable flash points and make mitigation plans, including for conflict resolution
- Celebrate every success in your consortium

Networks

- See your network is a long-term part of your career plan
- Look for opportunities for mutual advantage with network members
- At meetings or events be ready to invite people to join your network, for example, by using personal business cards
- Actively maintain contact with people in your network, for example, offering them updates about your work and achievements or links to new work that might be of interest to them
- Convert online to in-person meetings whenever you can
- Decide if you want to develop an operational, personal or strategic network (or hybrid)

Feedback

- We encourage you to actively seek, consider and use feedback
- In our view, learning is accelerated by using feedback
- Feedback is most useful if it focuses on particular behaviour and indicates specific ways to improve

- There is a range of types of feedback, including peer, downward, upward and coaching
- Particular techniques that can be helpful are 360-degree feedback, and audio- and video-recoding
- For students and trainees, feedback can be formative (during a course or module) or summative (testing at the end of a programme of teaching or learning)

References

Hardavella, G., Aamli-Gaagnat, A., Saad, N., Rousalova, I., & Sreter, K. B. (2017). How to give and receive feedback effectively. *Breathe (Sheff) 13*(4), 327–333.

Ibarra, H., & Hunter, M. (2017). How leaders create and use networks. *Harvard Bus. Rev 85*(1), 40–47. 124.

CHAPTER 29

How to Convince Others About the Usefulness of a Project

The remarks that follow here refer to projects that satisfy moral, legal and ethical requirements. Participation in projects that do not satisfy moral or legal requirements but serve ethically important causes often puts the person who undertakes them at risk of exclusion from society, blocks their career or their career development, or has even more dire consequences. This chapter will not deal with those.

Projects can be useful in two ways: they can result in a **product that will serve some worthwhile purpose**, for example, to provide information about the effectiveness and side-effects of a medication, or they can, regardless of their topic, **serve the person who has undertaken the project**, for example, in assisting in the process of promotion to a more attractive position in the hierarchy. Participating in a project usually serves both purposes, not necessarily equally well.

Convincing others that a project is useful will be easier and more effective if it can be shown that **there will be some specific and real benefit** (e.g., honoraria payments) for participants to take part in the project. The **benefit can be positive or negative**: positive if it increases income or helps in promotion, or negative if doing the work will help to avoid some unpleasant experience, task or consequence.

The probability that it will be possible to convince others to accept a suggestion increases if the leader has, in previous contact with them, **established the style of decision making** that they will use. There are several continua of decision making that will define the way in which one should approach those who are to be convinced.

Regarding decision-making styles, the first of these concerns the type of arguments that should be used in the conversation about the project. Some people will judge the proposal against principles that they consider important, whereas others tend to judge the attractiveness of a proposal on the basis of experience gained in previous work with similar proposals. Thus, if the proposal concerns engagement in a project that promotes a particular diet, the first group will start by seeking evidence that such a diet is useful for the purposes stated, while the other group will begin by seeking evidence that such projects have been successfully carried out in the group that is to be the target of the intervention. Knowing what decision style is typical for the team member who is to be convinced will help to formulate the argument and increase the probability that the proposal will be accepted.

A key task of the project leader is to **carefully select members of the team** to whom they will propose participation in the project. The selection should consider the **likely gains and losses for the individuals** who will be invited to participate in the project, as well as their personality features. Professional qualifications to participate in a project are usually of lesser importance than personal characteristics, because it is likely that the team members who will participate in the project will need to have **complementary skills** to serve the overall goal of the project.

Once the leader has selected the candidates on the grounds of their impression of the persons concerned, it will be necessary to **define and explain what their gains from participation would be** – expressing these in terms relevant to their personality, preferences and values.

Often it is likely that the **motivations for participation** in the project will vary among the team members. The task of the leader will be to motivate team members with reference to their personality, their value system, their previous experience and their capacity. The **enticement for participation must be personalised**, emphasising aspects of the project in harmony with the specific profile of each of the participants. Once the project has started, it will be important to maintain the motivation of participants. This again must be done by keeping the differences among the participants in mind.

The participants in the project team will also evaluate their experience, and temper their motivation to continue working on the basis of their perception of the satisfaction of their needs and values. The team leader's task will be to help the team members see the extent to which the participation in the **project satisfies their needs** and to **listen to their suggestions** about ways in which their satisfaction (and therefore their motivation to invest themselves) could be increased.

For the team leader, and for the other members of the team, it must be clear that well-designed and successful projects will result in **general and specific satisfaction** of the team members. The general satisfaction stems from the congruence of the project's goals and achievements with general ethical and humanitarian principles. The specific satisfaction depends on the personality, experience, value system and capacity of each of the team members, and will differ from one participant to another. The team leader should be aware of the individual differences and differing levels of satisfaction and motivation and ensure that the project contributes to both. If it does not, the team leader will have to invest time and energy to **create surrogate rewards** for the team members, whose motivation to participate may otherwise falter.

Key Points

- Projects can be useful because they serve some worthwhile purpose, or because they serve the person who has undertaken the project
- A team leader needs to convince a potential project team member that it will deliver to them some specific and real benefits (positive or negative)
- The leader needs to set the scene by establishing a clear **decision-making style**
- The team leader will also need to persuade team members with complementary skills to join the project
- The enticements for prospective team members can also be surrogate rewards offered by the team leader
- The benefits to each team member need to be general, and also personalised to be specific to their characters, values and needs

CHAPTER 30

How to Learn From the Failure of a Project

Whatever the setting of your work, sooner or later it is likely that you will be involved with, or perhaps even lead, a project that fails. This could be a proposal for a new team or service, a new course, or a research initiative. Whatever the specific details of the venture, how do you cope with such a failure? This chapter offers you some points to consider while trying to navigate one of the most difficult aspects of working life. Details of related chapters are shown below.

RELATED CHAPTERS

Chapter 16. How to lead a small working group or collaboration
Chapter 20. How to present a proposal for funding
Chapter 21. How to make an elevator pitch
Chapter 24. How to manage a poorly performing colleague
Chapter 26. How to reduce tension in a small group or in a meeting
Chapter 29. How to convince others about the usefulness of a project
Chapter 35. How to write a research paper
Chapter 42. How to admit an error or apologise

Project Failures at the Proposal Stage

The first point to make is that if you see a problem in your workplace or a way in which your efforts can be improved, or you want to see an innovation or initiative take place – *make a proposal*. For example, you may be a student where you feel that there is an important gap in the curriculum you are taught. Or you may be a junior professional where you are asked to fill in a time-consuming paper form that could be done much more efficiently online. Or you may be a junior researcher and you want to carry out an exciting new scientific project. In each case you could wait for someone else to take the initiative – and when this does not happen, you can of course complain bitterly. But much more useful is for you to contribute to a proposal for change. Perhaps your proposal may even be accepted.

Secondly, you will be more likely to succeed, and to enjoy developing a proposal if you *work in a team* (see Chapter 16). A small group will allow you to share the tasks, to learn from others, and to have a greater impact by making your proposal on behalf of a group rather than from one person alone. Nevertheless, especially in the field of research, most proposals fail, whether they are papers submitted to a scientific journal or grant applications for funds to conduct research. Is it possible to *cope with such repeated failures* and keep your morale high?

One technique we have found helpful is to try to separate criticism of your proposal from personal criticism of you as a person, that is, to *depersonalise the rejection*. In the field of science, the central process of quality assurance is peer review (see Chapter 35), and many journals and scientific funding bodies accept less than 10%, and sometimes fewer than 5%, of the proposals they receive. If you can take the rejection of a paper or a research proposal not to signal the end of this project, but as an opportunity to improve further what you are proposing, so much the better. This is easier to achieve if you have specific *feedback to use*. For a paper submitted to a journal, you may receive comments from reviewers that you can consider and use in revising the paper, and the same can apply to rejected grant applications. Core principles are to *keep revising the paper* and to keep improving it to the point where it will be accepted by a journal, and usually this will require subsequent submission to more modest journals, for example, as indicated by their impact factors.

Much more disappointing are situations where the journal or funding body rejects your proposal *without giving you any feedback*. In this case you may want to ask for comments from colleagues at work on how you can improve your initiative. For a paper, this will allow you to rewrite the paper to improve its chance of acceptance when submitted to an alternative journal. However, be *ready to abandon your project* proposal if you have consistent feedback, for example, from two or three experienced researchers whose opinions you trust, that the project is very unlikely to be improved to the level required to be fundable in competition with others in your field. In this case, have a debriefing session if you can on *what can be learned*, and move on to the next project idea.

If you are trying to improve an aspect of your organisation, for example, enhance a training curriculum or introduce an audit system to a clinical team, be less ready to give up on your idea. If the people higher up in your organisation do not accept your proposal, seek a *meeting to find out the reasons for their decision* and what changes to your plans could make the proposal acceptable. Wherever possible, try to find a way to *align your proposal* with the priorities and interests of the senior staff who can accept or reject your idea. Taking a conflictual stance to the authority figures in your organisation may not increase the likelihood of your success.

Projects That Fail During the Implementation Period

Situations in which projects or programmes are agreed and funded but then *fail to be completed* are less common but much more difficult to manage. There are many reasons why a project may fail midway through its planned period. For a *construction project*, there may be an unexpected increase in the costs of raw materials, a greater than expected inflation rate, or an unanticipated barrier in the supply of essential components. For a revision of a *teaching curriculum*, there can be the sudden departure of the programme manager, or a change of the strategic direction of the organisation because of a new senior leader. For a *clinical team*, there can be an unprecedented challenge to the core tasks, such as a major epidemic.

For a *research project*, there may be a catastrophic breakdown in relations between two or more of the senior staff. But a much more common reason for a *research project* to fail is that the initial calculations of the required number of *participants needing to be recruited* for the study were made purely on statistical calculations of power and sample size, without taking into account the realities of the numbers of people who would actually consent to take part in the study. Sometimes the remedy is to extend the recruitment period, but studies, especially randomised clinical trials, are surprisingly often abandoned for this reason.

Ways to *manage such failures* will vary in each case. In the construction example, alternative sources of supplies may be possible, or a revised timescale. Very often this depends on taking a *flexible approach in negotiating a project amendment with the project funder*. For the teaching curriculum illustration, the new or upgraded curriculum may need to subject to major or minor edits to fit into the new organisational priorities. For the clinical team, a proposal developed in more stable times may need to be paused or abandoned if a systemic challenge such as an epidemic has to be faced. In the research example, a revised recruitment sample size or project period may be acceptable to the funding body, but those providing oversight, often called the trial steering committee or the data monitoring and ethics committee, may conclude that the study is not viable and stop funding. In some cases the best form of *mitigation for these challenges* is prevention.

At the project design stage, produce a carefully considered list of *risks to the viability of the project*, and give concrete details of what can be done in advance to prevent or mitigate such risks (for example, appointing two rather than one person to lead specific project components, in case one leaves). Also add details of the anticipated action in case each risk does arise. The likelihood of successfully managing potentially fatal threats to the project are improved if the risks and their responses have been *identified in advance*.

If, despite your best efforts, a project is ended early, there are many difficult tasks to undertake. You may have to *terminate the employment contracts* for some or all staff. This will be somewhat less traumatic for the staff if you have communicated to them in advance the possibility of project failure, but this is difficult to do without some staff concluding that they should *move on to other posts* immediately, and their loss can itself undermine the viability of the work. You may need to finalise reports and budgets of the partially complete work after the project staff have left. There may be reputational damage to you if the work is seen within your own organisation to have failed because of your incompetence, so you need to *communicate early, regularly and clearly with your managers and senior staff* what is happening and why, and how you are managing the difficult situation very well. It is vital to communicate clearly both with junior project staff and with the project funders, and with senior staff in your organisation if severe problems arise, and *tell them what you plan to do and how they can assist you*. This is also true if you are working on a project where some of the tasks *fall behind their intended timetable* and deadlines are not met. It is important in this case to have very *clear milestones* (intermediate deadlines leading to the completion of a task) and to *identify at an early stage* when progress on a particular talk is too slow. The project coordinator needs to make an early identification of any delays and to *intervene quickly* to provide practical support to accelerate catch up with the agreed timetable, or to *renegotiate the time plan*. For research projects, for example, a very common problem is that the *recruitment of study participants* takes place much more slowly than anticipated. Early intervention is vital: first to understand the reasons for slow progress, and then to apply practical measures to remedy the shortfall.

In this worst-case scenario, you are likely to be very busy for weeks or months if you have to close down a project early. If you can, after a pause, try to make time to *reflect with colleagues*, to calmly talk through what happened and why it happened. Were steps in the terminal sequence of events predictable or preventable? Could you have reacted earlier? Did you recruit all the support you could have to avert project closure? In short, what can you *learn to improve your future project management skills*?

Projects That End and Are Not Sustained

A much more common situation is where a programme, for example, a clinical team or a research project, receives funding for a fixed period and is then not sustained. One of us, for example, worked with a team of colleagues to *initiate a new clinical team* for people of a black and minoritised ethnic group with depression. The innovative aspect of this project was that the team staff were black, to make the clinical support more acceptable to the service users. Despite evidence from a randomised clinical trial that this service was effective, the team was only continued for a short period by the local mental health service provider and was cut when the health services entered a period of economic austerity. Indeed, it is our experience that most clinical service innovations that are evaluated in research projects (where their effectiveness or cost effectiveness is assessed) are closed when the research funding ends.

Can the *failure of project sustainability be anticipated and prevented*? Perhaps, but not very often. For health service innovations, it can help, at the start of the project, to *bring into the group of project stakeholders, senior staff from local health provider or health commissioner organisations* who you will later approach to continue funding the service if it is a success. Even so, the results of the evaluation may appear 3–5 years after the start of the project and, commonly, health service funders find it difficult or impossible to commit funds in their budgets more than a year ahead. Another approach is to *include among the stakeholders service user and family representatives*. These groups recognise that it is in their direct best interests to have more effective services provided locally, and if they are involved with the project, preferably also from the very start of the work, they can advocate for continuation funding to be provided if the final evaluation of the project is that it delivers benefits to its patients or clients.

Finally, if you are a part of a team managing a project failure, especially if you are the team leader, expect to find this an *extremely stressful time in your life*. Remember the basics of physical exercise and fitness, pay attention to getting enough rest and sleep, try to maintain a healthy diet, do not work all the time, make space for time with friends and family, and share the duties of managing the project closure with a team that supports one another.

Personal Factors Associated With Projects

As well as project management-related factors, the successful completion of a project can be affected by much more *personal factors*. For example, you or your partner may choose or need to *move to a different city* or country for your work. Even in the age of remote and hybrid working, if you have an important responsibility for the project, your relocation or your new work duties may mean that you are not able to continue to be involved in the project until its completion. The best response to such a situation is to *foresee and mitigate* for this in advance. For example, each module or work package in a project could have *two lead staff* allocated from the start of the project (as long as they collaborate well with each other). This *gives a project some degree of reserve or redundancy* so that if one in the module leaves, there is still one knowledgeable lead to continue this part of the work. In a similar way, you may have periods of *illness or family illness* that reduce your ability to completely fulfil your project responsibilities. Such events occur frequently among members of a project team. *Advance planning* also helps to mitigate the impact of these occurrences. Such discontinuities are, however, also *opportunities for junior staff* in a project group to step up, at least temporarily, into a more senior role. If other members of the group can *provide close support* to the temporarily responsible person, these events can in fact be very *valuable opportunities for accelerated learning*, as long as the role is feasible, and as long as support to the junior person is strong and reliable.

A less positive challenge to project teams and their ability to complete projects can happen when there is a *serious breakdown in the working relationship* between key team members. This can occur either between existing staff, or when a new member of staff joins the team. The first step can be for the project coordinator to invite the conflicting or warring parties to *informally discuss their disagreement* and to find agreement, for example, make a compromise. The second step is for the *project leader to mediate* by meeting, preferably in person, between the staff who have personal friction. In this case the project leader will need to *listen carefully* to both sides, to understand both differences and agreements of perspective, and to *invite proposals* for partial or full solutions. This may take some time if both sides feel that they are misunderstood or being wronged, with periods of reflection between meetings. If no compromise can be found, then it may be necessary for the team leader to reluctantly invite one or both of those who cannot agree to *leave the project team*, so that the project can make progress towards completion.

Key Points

- If you are dissatisfied with an aspect of your work, make a proposal for change, preferable working with a team
- For project failures at the proposal stage, try to depersonalise the rejection, seek feedback and discuss how to make future proposals better
- For a scientific paper, persist, revise the paper and submit to a more modest journal
- For a workplace innovation, seek the advice of senior colleagues and be prepared either to revise the proposal to align with the current priorities of senior staff, or to drop the proposal if the view of people you trust is that the project is not viable
- Take a flexible approach in negotiating a project amendment with the project funder
- Try to avoid preventable problems by identifying risks to the project at the design stage and listing measures to prevent, mitigate or manage any risk that does occur
- Communicate clearly with the junior project staff, funders and senior staff in your organisation if severe problems arise and tell them what you plan to do and how they can assist you
- If you do need to close a project, support your senior team during this stressful period and debrief later to see what can be learned
- To improve the likelihood of a project being sustained after its initial funding period, include the potential future project funders in your stakeholder group from the very start of the project, and include service user and family members, who may become strong advocates for the project in the future

CHAPTER 31

How to Work Well in Video and Online Collaborations

The COVID-19 pandemic in 2020–2023 transformed how many people worldwide communicate with each other. For example, many clinical and research teams almost immediately used remote, online and telemedicine methods of communication to a far greater extent than had been usual before the pandemic. Several other chapters in this book, shown below, cover related aspects such as working well in small groups and using technology, especially video meetings. In this chapter we supplement those chapters by focusing specifically on how to to effectively make the most of video and online methods of collaborating with colleagues.

RELATED CHAPTERS

Chapter 7. How to overcome language problems
Chapter 8. How to work with people from other cultures
Chapter 12. How to prepare for a meeting
Chapter 14. How to take part in a meeting
Chapter 16. How to lead a small working group or collaboration
Chapter 19. How to take part in a video meeting
Chapter 25. How to work in a small group

The Major Differences Between In-Person and Online Contact

In our experience, there are several major differences between in-person and online meetings. Firstly, it is more difficult to ***get to know other colleagues and to build trust in your relationship*** using online meetings. We find that once you have met a new person directly and if you have started to build a reasonable or good working relationship, video-meeting later can extend the collaboration. But never having met the other in person tends to limit the sense of how well you know the person. In part this is because video meetings tend to filter out most of the more subtle nonverbal signals from the other person, but also because at in-person meetings you can take the opportunity of quiet moments before or after meetings, or during drink or meal breaks, to find out more about other people and their families and backgrounds.

Secondly, we find that in-person meetings are far more effective at *managing or solving the tensions, difficulties and conflicts* that often arise within a working group or collaboration. If you are in the position of having to mediate between colleagues who disagree on an issue, or even when you have a conflict with a colleague, it can be very difficult to assess online the strength of their feelings or sometimes to clarify precisely the point of disagreement. We find that arranging to meet in person, if necessary, for one-to-one discussions is usually a better way to resolve conflicts.

Another downside of online meetings is that it is harder to *assess the health, status and morale of colleagues*. In a larger consortium there will always be some colleagues who are flourishing in their lives and some who are languishing. The collaboration is likely to be more effective if at least some in the group, usually the leaders or coordinators, know who may be struggling, for example, because of work or home life pressures, and to take this into account, for example, by not loading extra tasks and pressures on this person during a time of stress.

In terms of your organisation, in-person meetings make it easier to *gather soft knowledge and background intelligence* about what is happening or about to happen, for example, staff who have been promoted or who are going to leave their posts, or other useful gossip. This may be useful to know in terms of who is becoming more or less powerful within your or other organisations.

Online and remote meetings bring a further difficulty, because project or team leaders will find it *harder to identify delays or difficulties in the tasks that need to be completed* at an early stage. We have found that in-person meetings are more likely to allow quiet conversations in which a person who is failing to deliver a task can mention this at an early stage, when the problem is easier to fix. Online meetings, by comparison, more often do not allow discreet conversations and a person who is not delivering their work may be too embarrassed to be open about this to the whole group, so that when the problem is identified at a later stage, it has become worse and more complex, and will be harder to solve.

A final challenge for online meetings that we have encountered is that it is more difficult to create an atmosphere in which the *group goes into a creative 'brainstorm' mode* or mood. In this mode the usual hierarchies and power relationships can be temporarily or partially suspended, so that the creative potential within the group is sparked with a rapid-fire round of ideas, some of which will be valuable. This tends to work well when the group have already 'bonded' and built some degree of trust in each other, when the group or session leaders create a spirit in which ideas will not be criticised or sanctioned, and where the session becomes one that participants enjoy. All of these characteristics tend to be harder to achieve online than in person.

Mitigating the Effects of Losing In-Person Contact

Given these challenges, how can you minimise the disadvantages of working online? We suggest a series of practical steps. Firstly, there is an additional responsibility for the team leader or coordinator to *be very clear about what is expected of each group* or team member, communicated, for example, during video meetings or via email or other electronic forms. Be sure to pass on papers for meetings well in advance, for example, a week ahead, so group members can prepare for the meeting if they want to. Those chairing online meetings are less able to assess the feelings of participants than at in-person meetings, and may need to more formally *ask whether group members agree with particular proposals* or provisional decisions. Where this is possible, *hybrid arrangements* can help a group to function well, for example, a committee that meets every 3 months may have two or three meetings online, and one or two meetings in person, to greet new members and to have time for lunch or an evening meal together. Similarly, a project group that meets every month can have 10–11 meetings each year online and one or two meetings in person to recognise the social dimension of good interpersonal communication and collaboration.

Optimising the Benefits of Online Contact

There are also several clear benefits to online group working. Apart from the subscription fee for a video meeting programme and the costs of the time of participants, such *meetings can be essentially cost free*. As an example, these authors contributed to The Lancet Commission on Ending Stigma and Discrimination in Mental Health (Thornicroft et al., 2022), and, because this was written during the COVID-19 pandemic, the 50 or so colleagues across the world who contributed to this report never met and no funds were required for the consortium to complete its work. The low cost nature of online meetings means that *more frequent meetings* can be arranged, or meetings at short notice when urgent issues arise. *Jet lag and contributions to climate change* and global warming are also minimised. Indeed, video meetings can *release parts of a team or project budget* for other purposes, such as allowing junior colleagues fees for training opportunities or payment for academic processing charges for journal papers. Online meetings can also produce *large savings in time lost* to travelling and the stress and fatigue of negotiating traffic, train stations or airports.

We also find several other advantages to online meetings. Quiet or modest colleagues who speak quietly and who can be hard to hear at in-person meetings are often *more audible online*. The *share screen option* in many video programmes means that *documents can be easily shared during meetings, and edited live*, for example, when colleagues at different sites update the whole group on progress with project tasks. These video programmes can also *automatically manage time zone differences* and periods when clocks change on different dates in the spring and autumn. Additional facilities are chat comments for smaller groups, question and answer options for larger gatherings, and the ability to *record video meetings* to help others to see the meeting later and to assist the person making a record of the meeting. For larger occasions, smaller *break-out groups* are easy to organise.

If you are leading online meetings, be aware that the *technologies are often variable*, for example, with time lags before people can comment, or fluctuating quality of sound or vision, and do ask participants to speak slowly and clearly and with a great deal of consideration for one another. Tend to have short and frequent breaks, for example 5–10 minutes every hour, to allow people at the meeting to retain focus on the work. Even deliberately ask if the group members need a break, or prefer to actively move ahead to the end of the meeting.

For meetings of people from across the world, video technology allows, for example, the duplication of meetings on the same topic for the *western and eastern hemispheres* at convenient times, although reconciling can be problematic if the two groups disagree with each other! For a process such a *Delphi exercise* to move towards consensus on a topic, video meetings can work well, for example, with rapid rounds of voting using 'raise hand' to come to a shared view on an issue, such as a clinical recommendation or guideline. There are now many online *'whiteboard' apps* that can be linked to video conferencing programs to allow groups to work together to make suggestions, prioritise ideas and converge on agreements.

An important advantage of online meetings is that they can radically *promote wider participation and inclusion*. For example, people who cannot afford the travel, accommodation and meeting registration costs, such as for an international conference, may find that an online option is free or affordable. This will particularly apply to patients, service users and family members, as well as colleagues working in low- and middle-income countries.

Key points

- Keep in mind that there are several clear advantages to in-person meetings, such as getting to know colleagues, building trust and resolving conflicts
- In-person meetings allow you to know more about the morale and wellbeing of colleagues and to gather background soft information about what is happening in your organisation
- In-person meetings can allow team or project delays or challenges to be identified earlier
- There are many advantages to online meetings, including cost saving and reducing time spent travelling
- The features of online video meetings confer a number of benefits, such as the use of chat and question and answer functions; the ability to record meetings, share screens and update documents live; and the ability to make meetings suitable for different time zones
- The low costs of video meetings can radically promote wider participation and inclusion in meetings and projects

Reference

Thornicroft, G., Sunkel, C., Alikhon Aliev, A., Baker, S., Brohan, E., et al., (2022). The Lancet Commission on ending stigma and discrimination in mental health. *Lancet, 400*(10361), 1438–1480.

Skills Needed to Work Well Alone

In this third main section of the book, the frame of reference becomes smaller still. Here we focus on important skills that will enable you to be more effective in working alone. For career purposes, one important ability is promoting yourself to others using a compelling curriculum vitae, accompanied by an engaging letter of motivation. If you are interested in using or creating research, the chapters on how to read and write scientific papers and how to choose a research topic may be informative. Whatever your specific role or profession, the overarching and lifelong questions of how to decide on your priorities in life and how to manage your precious time are likely to preoccupy you, and so we offer information and advice on these pressing issues here.

We appreciate that you will have different preferences and characteristics to other readers of this book. You may have to adapt some of our advice to align with the approaches that work best for you in dealing with the challenges we describe. Nevertheless, we endeavour to provide information about skills that may well be valid in the scenarios described in these chapters, regardless of your specific circumstances and existing skills.

CHAPTER 32

How to Write a Curriculum Vitae/Resume

What Is a CV/Resume?

A curriculum vitae, called a resume in some countries and a CV in this chapter, is an outline of a person's educational and professional history. It is usually prepared for job applications but can have other uses. The phrase originates in Latin, meaning '*the course (or the running) of one's life*'. Related chapters are show below.

RELATED CHAPTERS

Chapter 10. How to present oneself to a group of people
Chapter 18. How to behave in an interview for a post
Chapter 21. How to make an elevator pitch
Chapter 33. How to write a letter of motivation (cover letter)
Chapter 37. How to apply for a post

Why Make a CV?

A CV is a **marketing document** – you are marketing yourself! It is a document that can be useful when you need to 'sell' your skills, abilities, qualifications and experience, for example, to an employer.

It should be appreciated that a CV is not a general document; rather, each version of an individual's CV **should be *specific* to a particular situation or job application**. For example, the content for a particular CV should be deliberately selected to be directly relevant to a specific work opportunity, and so be different from other versions of a person's CV.

A common purpose of a CV is **to get a job interview**. Often job applications will first have a written stage, and second have an interview stage. The CV may be part of the application used by an employer to choose who to interview. Sometimes the CV is the only document used to shortlist who to interview.

Although a CV should be made specific to each separate occasion or job application, we strongly suggest that you **make a master version of your CV**, complete with your full details, which you regularly update, for example, every month or two, so that you can easily take material from this for each particular shorter version of your CV that you need to prepare.

WHEN TO USE A CV

Use a CV when an employer asks to see your CV as part of a recruitment process. If the length or the format preferred by the employer is not specified, **ask for further details**. In particular, if an employer wants only a short CV, for example, two pages, do not send a much longer version. A CV can also be used for a **speculative approach** to a potential future employer, for example, if you want to work for a particular company but you have not seen any relevant vacancies advertised. In this case you can write to a specific key person in the organisation, sending them your CV, with a covering letter (see below) to make it clear why you are sending your CV. This could say, for example, that you greatly admire or respect the work of the company and that you are aware of their fine reputation, or it could give another positive reason for your approach. It would also ask them to keep your details on file should any relevant opening be available in future.

The Main Sections of a CV

The format of CVs varies a great deal in different settings and contexts. Generally a CV will have the following sections:

Personal identifiers: name and contact information. In our view, it is wise to put less detail here if the CV is to be posted to a public or semipublic domain such an internet CV repository. This section will often include:

- Name
- Address
- Phone contact number
- Date of birth
- Nationality
- Postal address

Your contact details. Make sure that these are current. You may be offered a job at short notice, for example, if you are a stand-by candidate, and the employer must be able to reach you quickly.

In some sectors it is customary to include a short *summary statement*, for example, stating 'I am an excellent communicator who works well in a team…' or 'I would like to work in a humanitarian international organisation and would enjoy challenges such as coordinating, information management, public health communications and engaging with multiple sectors to achieve goals.' Our preference is not to include such a generic introductory statement but rather to include your key strengths within the body of the CV.

Education and qualifications: Where and when you studied, and which qualifications you have completed. If you are later offered a particular job or position, the employer may ask for certified copies of these qualifications, so be sure that this information is complete and accurate. Included here may be details of:

- postgraduate study
- first degree or other university/college qualifications
- school qualifications

Work experience: It is common to format this section in reverse chronological order, that is, to show your most recent experience first and then to list work experience backwards in time in the following sections. Emphasise your more recent and relevant experience. Details of periods of paid employment are included here, and any periods of unpaid work that are directly relevant to this job. If there are particular time gaps in your record of employment, think carefully about giving enough information to explain why your employment has not been continuous.

Skills: The key issue for this section is to focus on the skills you have that are directly relevant to the post being advertised. If the job description says that having a driving licence is a required criterion for a particular post, or is an advantage for this post, then say if you have such a licence. In other words, clearly state in your CV information that will allow the employer to quickly assess if you meet enough of the job requirements to be able to shortlist you for an interview.

Emphasise transferrable skills, that is, capabilities you have developed in previous posts that you can use in future employment positions. These will depend on the specific type of occupation but may include, for example, information technology skills, languages used, or specific technical knowledge. Wherever possible, give specific detail about your proficiency level, for example, accredited examination levels or grades. If you state a given level of language proficiency, be aware that the interview may, at least in part, be held in that language to test this skill.

Interests, achievements and personal characteristics: Employers or directors of training activities are very unlikely to be interested in the fact that you like to cook or watch films in your spare time, or to travel during your vacations, unless this is directly relevant to the particular posts for which you are applying. However, if you have led a group of explorers to a remote and dangerous mountain top amid atrocious weather, and show exceptional ingenuity or adaptability amid dangerous challenges, you may wish to refer to such experience, if you can directly connect such achievements with skills you will need for this particular job. Keep in mind here the need to directly show relevance.

Referees: A CV will often have a section at or near the end for referees. This will often give the names and contact details of two or three senior people who know you and your recent work well and who you are confident will give you, if asked, a positive report. Only include the name and details of a person if you have their prior permission to do so, usually for a particular application for a specific post. Ask senior colleagues you have worked with fairly recently, for example, in the last year or two, not people with whom you worked 5 or 10 years ago. Treat your referees very kindly and let them know how you are and what you are doing from time to time, particularly thanking them for assisting with your career progression. Sometimes, to avoid referees being contacted too often, you may add at the end of your CV that you will make referees' details available to an employer at a later stage in the application process, for example, at interview, or if you are offered the position. Be sure that the contact details, such as the email or phone numbers, for your referees are current and active. One of the referees should be linked to your current employment.

How Long Should the CV Be?

Often employers will not make clear how long a CV should be. If in doubt, ask. If you cannot get information about CV length, as a general guide, for a first contact with an employer make your CV two pages; for an academic or technical position, four or five pages; and for a senior position, a much longer CV is required with all your relevant strengths over the course of your career.

How to Format and Present Your CV

- Use a clear and consistent common font style that is not flamboyant.
- Use a consistent font and font size (usually 11- or 12-point) for the whole CV.
- Use only black font or a very limited number of colours, for example, for headings and subheadings.
- Avoid all abbreviations or acronyms that may not be clear to all your target CV readers.
- Carefully proofread the CV for spelling errors, which give a very bad impression to employers. One study found that compared with CVs with spelling errors, those with no spelling mistakes led to 61% more replies and 26% more interviews.

It is common to include dates for the most important qualifications and periods of relevant employment. Make sure all the parts of your CV stress your positive aspects and your strengths – usually do not include any self-critical comments or reference to any of your limitations. Be sure that all the information you include in your CV is honest and accurate. If you are applying for a job in another country, or even in a sector in your own country with which you are not familiar, take time to learn the usual format used for a CV in that country or that sector.

Commonly made mistakes in CVs include the following:

- Using humour to try to make a good impression. Humour can easily go wrong so it is best to avoid any jokes or witty comments in a CV.
- Being overfamiliar in the content of the CV. It is wiser to recognise the CV as a part of a formal process of recruitment and to show a high level of respect to future readers of your CV.
- Using a mixture of fonts, dramatic font and/or variation in font sizes and colours – keep font use simple and consistent.

- Arranging some sections in forward and some sections in backward chronological order – decide on one time format and keep to it for all sections of the CV, unless your instructions tell you to do otherwise.
- Forgetting to include your current and accurate contact details.
- Including out-of-date information, for example, for the contact details of your referees.
- Including inappropriate details, for example, the name of the last organisation you applied to.
- Including an old date at the front of the CV, showing that you have not updated it recently.
- Including notes to yourself in the CV such as (this section to be updated).
- Including general information such as Dear Sir/Madam in your covering letter rather than the actual name of the specific person to whom the CV needs to be sent.

Example of a Bad CV

CV section	CV content	Commentary
Title	Dr (name)	<ul><li>No organisational address at the top of the CV and no alternative contact address</li><li>No email contact</li><li>No phone contact</li></ul>
Personal information	Married with three children	<ul><li>No date of birth or age</li><li>Details of partner and children not relevant</li></ul>
Qualifications	Qualified from medical school	<ul><li>No dates of qualifications</li><li>No name for medical school</li><li>No details of further qualifications</li></ul>
Experience	Various medical roles in a number of hospitals	<ul><li>No detail about the roles</li><li>No details about the types of experience</li><li>No details about skills gained, or where or when</li></ul>
Personal interests	I love to travel I am passionate about cooking. In my spare time I like to watch movies on Netflix I have a pet cat at home called Fluff	<ul><li>None of this is relevant for the post being applied for</li><li>Only include information about personal interests if it is directly relevant to this particular post</li></ul>

Social Media

Social media or CV libraries can easily make your details available either publicly or to a wide online audience. **Think carefully** before you decide to include, for example, your home address or your private phone number, bearing in mind that strangers may have access to this. Also ask yourself, is there *any* information in the public domain, for example, on social media sites, that could compromise your future applications for jobs? Pictures of you being less than sober or comments by you that could be taken out of context might be examined by organisations, and could harm your employment opportunities. Also check to see if there is any information in the public domain that is not consistent with what you include in your CV, such as details of your education or qualifications.

Key Points

- Keep a regularly updated master version of your CV
- Each particular of your CV should be prepared for a specific purpose
- In each particular version, only include information relevant to each application
- Be sure to check important details such as contact details for you and your referees
- Spend time writing a strong and short cover letter (letter of motivation)
- Ask friends or close colleagues to comment on your draft CV and cover letter
- From the feedback you get, aim to make your next CV and cover letter even better

CHAPTER 33

How to Write a Letter of Motivation

In recent times, applications for posts or requests to attend meetings are usually submitted in writing, providing the organiser with all the necessary documents and adding a 'letter of motivation,' which is often called a 'covering letter'. This chapter discusses how to construct a strong letter of motivation.

Such a letter sets out: (1) reasons **why the applicant wishes to be selected** for the post or stipend; and (2) the **special skills** or other attributes that are usually not covered in the curriculum vitae or not covered in enough detail. Letters of motivation are meant to provide these two sets of information in an easy-to-read style. The letter will usually have **four key sections**: an introduction, a statement of reasons for applying, a statement of skills or other assets supporting the application, and a closing summary paragraph. The introduction will state to whom the application is sent (by name) and for what purpose. Both statements are important because they will make it easy to **link the letter to the other documents** relevant to the application, in case they get separated.

The second paragraph will state **why the candidate is applying** for this post. In this paragraph the applicant should not put themselves forward; thus the statement should not end by saying that the candidate will improve his skills (if this is a course, for example). Rather, it should **say what the candidate will do better in his job,** for example, that they will be **provide better care** to a specific group of patients who need to be treated using the skills that the course will provide – or that they **will teach others** who need this knowledge. To write the paragraph convincingly, it is important to **study the invitation carefully** to discover specific improvements of capacity that could be expected from the training that will be received on the course.

The third paragraph should contain **specific characteristics of the candidate** that make them **likely to gain maximum benefit from the training** that will be offered. Here again, to write convincingly it is important to be specific, stating which of the characteristics and what knowledge or previous experience of the candidate is likely to make a difference.

To write a good letter of motivation it is important to be **well informed about the object of the application** and the **expectations of the host** who invited applications. Once the characteristics of the recipient and the characteristics of their achievements are clear, it is possible to include in the letter an **indication of links between these achievements and the ambition of the applicant**. We end this chapter with examples of poor and good letters of motivation.

Examples of **poor and good letters of motivation** are shown in Table 33.1, along with a commentary.

Key Points

- The letter of motivation will usually include: (1) the reasons why the applicant wishes to be selected for the post; and (2) the special skills or other attributes that the applicant brings
- The letter will contain four key sections: an introduction, a statement of reasons for applying, a statement of skills or other assets supporting the application, and a closing summary paragraph
- The letter can usefully summarise why a particular job or training course will support the applicant to better help others
- The letter needs to be specific to the job or other opportunity that is being applied for
- Address the letter to the relevant named person

TABLE 33.1 ■ **Poor and Good Examples of Letters of Motivation**

Paragraph	Poor Example	Good Example	Commentary
1	Dear Sir or Madam, With this letter, I should like to express my interest in participating in your course on Leadership and Professional skills for early career psychiatrists.	Dear Professor Masterson, I am writing in relation to the announcement that you will direct a course on Leadership and Professional Skills in Zagreb on 16–18 December 2017.	■ Address the letter to a specific, named person ■ Give the specific details of the event with place and date ■ Write directly in relation only to this specific event ■ Do not use the same letter for more than one event
2	My name is Dr Max Cleverley and I am a third-year resident in our psychiatric department. Personally, I think of myself as a proactive individual, avid about psychiatry, always willing to maintain an optimal performance at work, and continuously eager to improve my skills. I can contribute with my proven eagerness to learn, active participation and intensive focus. The desire to learn new skills that are useful to others drives and motivates me. I am a worthy and responsible person with much interest and desirability to implement my ambitions. I am not afraid of challenges in spite of marked individuality. My presence at your course would undoubtedly contribute to the course quality.	I am very keen to attend this course. I heard about its contents and method of work from colleagues in my country and elsewhere. They were enthusiastic in their descriptions, pointing out that they have learned a lot and that the skills that they have acquired have not been taught to them ever before.	■ Give the proper name of your department ■ Avoid unnecessary or incomprehensible words such as 'proactive' ■ 'Always willing' may suggest that the person in fact fails in this respect ■ Avoid exaggerated or self-aggrandising statements about yourself ■ 'Marked individuality' can suggest you are self-centred and difficult to work with ■ Do not specify your contribution to the course in advance – others will make this judgement after the course ■ Do refer to the sources of information you are using ■ Do indicate that you have examined the course programme and you know what you expect to learn

(Continued)

TABLE 33.1 ■ Poor and Good Examples of Letters of Motivation—cont'd

Paragraph	Poor Example	Good Example	Commentary
3	I already applied for this course in Türkiye, and I was selected. Unfortunately, I was simultaneously accepted by a course in neuropsychopharmacology organised by ECNP in Oxford that took place at the same time. For pragmatic reasons, I decided to take the CINP course. The course at Oxford was a very pleasant and enriching experience, for the knowledge acquired and the opportunity to exchange experiences and meet young psychiatrists from all parts of the world.	My current position as a third-year resident in the department of psychiatry of the Medical School in Vilnius requires that I give talks to medical and nursing students and that I make presentations at scientific meetings in my country. Improving my presentation skills – which I know would happen if I attended your course – would make my teaching better and render me more useful to my department and to my colleagues.	■ Do not say that you think the course is a second-best option for you ■ Do not include irrelevant information in your letter ■ Do not suggest that you are unprincipled, deviously pragmatic or self-serving ■ Do say how you will use the knowledge you will learn on the course – importantly, for the benefit of others
4	In parallel with my training programme I joined a private psychotherapeutic practice in *******, where I work passionately with different types of patients. Finally, I have never participated in any of your skill training courses, and I am very curious about it. My attendance at this training is a wise investment and I would highly appreciate to be one of the selected participants.	The other skills mentioned in the description of the course are also central to my work and I would therefore be very glad to attend your course. I would of course undertake any preparatory work for the course that you might wish us to do.	■ 'Wise investment' is ambiguous, but sounds as if the applicant is selfish ■ Do say that you are happy to undertake preparatory work to make attendance at the course more rewarding, and to show your willingness to do what is necessary for successful participation in the course

Paragraph	Poor Example	Good Example	Commentary
5	You may write to me if you need more information and I shall reply as soon as my other professional and personal obligations permit me to do so.	There are two more reasons for my applying and for hoping that I shall be selected to attend the course. The first is that the course would give me an opportunity to meet you and learn directly from you. I have read several papers that you have published and admired their clarity and relevance to clinical practice and applied research: it would be a great privilege to meet you in person and attend your teachings. The second reason is that I hope that the course will give me opportunities to meet colleagues of my age and level of seniority with whom I might collaborate and from whom I could also learn. Vilnius can be a lonely place for a trainee in psychiatry and contacts with my peers are a precious commodity for me.	■ As the applicant, do not suggest that you are in a superior position to the course organiser ■ Do not say how busy you are ■ Avoid flattery and sycophantic comments (overly lavish praise for the teacher) ■ Do state any additional benefits of your attending the course, such as forming and developing your social and professional networks ■ Do say a little about your personal or emotional reasons for wanting to attend the course
6	I look forward to hearing from you in the near future. Sincerely	My curriculum vitae lists my address but I am listing it below to make it easier to ensure that I can be reached immediately should additional information be necessary.	■ Do not tell the course organiser they must reply rapidly ■ Do imagine yourself as the course organiser, and make it easy for them to select you. For example, give your contact details clearly so it is easy to contact you

CHAPTER 34

How to Read a Research Paper

During your years training in your post or your profession you will need to decide whether you want to spend time reading research papers in your field. This chapter helps you to navigate this question. Related chapters are shown below.

Should You Read, and What Should You Read, During Your Training?

There are several **reasons for reading papers** during your training.

- To be **informed** about the subjects of importance to your profession.
- To **keep track of what your friends** and superiors are publishing so you can talk with them about it.
- To **learn what can be published** and in which type of journal.
- To be **informed about developments in health care** in general – for example, by reading a general medical journal with a high impact factor and a general medical journal published in your own country.
- To assess the **trends in your field**, for example, towards a greater focus on biological investigations or a new and growing emphasis on social factors or social care.

In the biomedical field alone, each year more than a million papers describing findings of research are published and added to the PubMed database – about two papers every minute. You may be active in undertaking research or in collaborating in research projects, and in this case you are likely to want to keep up to date with your particular field of enquiry. You may be early in your clinical or social care career and be interested to see what papers are being published by your colleagues or friends. You may be thinking about getting involved in research and exploring which questions seem to have been answered by recent published research and which questions still need to be answered. You may have been involved with an interesting or complex case or client recently and want to know how to treat or support the person using the most recent evidence. There are many reasons why you may want to read research papers, but how do you start?

Starting Your Search

The first step is usually to **arrange access to an online database or library**, and for health-related research a useful starting point is PubMed, the searchable version of the National Library of Medicine in the United States (https://pubmed.ncbi.nlm.nih.gov/). You will see that you can enter one or more 'terms' to search for papers. A 'term' can be the name of an author, the name of a condition (such as bipolar disorder), a type of research design (such as 'randomised controlled trial'), a type of paper (such as 'systematic review') or a year of publication. You can also combine terms, for example, 'systematic review', 'Alzheimer's' and 'cognition'.

To guide you through the search process, let us imagine that you are working in a unit specialising in the treatment of people with eating disorders, such as anorexia or bulimia. You want to know if the risk factors for eating disorders for young women are the same as for young men. Within the PubMed website, if you use the 'advanced search' option you can combine several search terms, for example, 'eating', 'disorder', 'risk', and 'factor', and then press 'search'. See Chapter 39 for more details about how to search for information.

Assessing the Paper Title

The results of the search will probably be a display of paper summaries, showing paper authors, title, year of publication and journal. Your **first task is to check the paper titles** to find papers that are of interest to you. These will be located by the database search as papers that include your search terms either in the title of the paper or in the 'key words' of the paper. Key words are a few words that are included in the paper, usually on the first page, that are provided by the paper's authors to help people locate this paper in future literature searches.

Your next decision is whether, from looking at the paper's title, you **want to spend any more time on this paper or not**. Can you understand the title? Does it stimulate your curiosity? Does the title suggest that the content of the papers is about the topic that you want to explore? If not, drop this paper. If you have positive responses to some of these questions, the next step is to go to the paper abstract. In PubMed you do this simply by clicking on the paper title, and this will usually take you to the paper abstract. See Chapter 36 for more details about the titles of research papers.

Reading the Paper Abstract

The **abstract of a research paper** is written by the paper authors with the aim of giving a brief and clear summary, often in 150–250 words, of the full paper. The format of the abstract varies somewhat for different journals, but it usually includes background, methods, results and discussion. As you read the abstract, ask the same questions as you did about the paper title. There are three options after you have read the abstract: drop the paper; note the paper, if the information in the abstract is enough for you; or go to the full paper. If the abstract is not relevant to your search, or relevant but incomprehensible, then drop the paper. If you find the abstract is relevant and is so clearly written that you can gather the main issue addressed and the key findings simply from the abstract itself, then make a note of the paper and then move on to the next title. If the abstract is probably about your core interest but is not clear enough, or if it is directly and highly relevant to your search and you want more details of the study, then go further to retrieve the full paper. This will usually be much simpler if you can access the main paper via a university or health care organisation login or credentials, which allow free access to the full papers of many journals.

Reading the Main Paper

One way to read a research paper is to think of it as a **short story**. The start of the story is usually a question. Does the paper state the aims of the project that it reports? Does it state these aims clearly? Are there just a few aims of the study, or preferably just one? Is this stated as a question? Do you find the central question interesting, important, or preferably both? As you read the paper do you have a sense of 'flow' whereby each section leads clearly to the next as the story unfolds? Can you understand every stage of the research inquiry being described? Do the decisions taken by the study authors, such as which research design to use, seem reasonable and well justified to you? Is the paper written to be clearly understandable for readers whose first language is not English? Are sentences and paragraphs long or (preferably) short? Is there limited use of abbreviations and acronyms? Can you easily navigate the paper, for example, because there are clear and helpful headings and subheadings? If you find a paper hard to understand, you may want to save it, and then come back to that paper after you have read more basic papers in that field and you understand the main concepts more clearly.

There are now internationally agreed **conventions on how to report the methods and results** of particular types of research study. Many journals will not consider these types of paper unless they conform to these guidelines, and details of many of these guidelines are available at https://www.equator-network.org/reporting-guidelines/:

- CONSORT guidelines for reporting randomised controlled trials
- STROBE for reporting observational studies
- MOOSE for reporting meta-analyses
- PRISMA for reporting systematic reviews
- COREQ for reporting qualitative studies

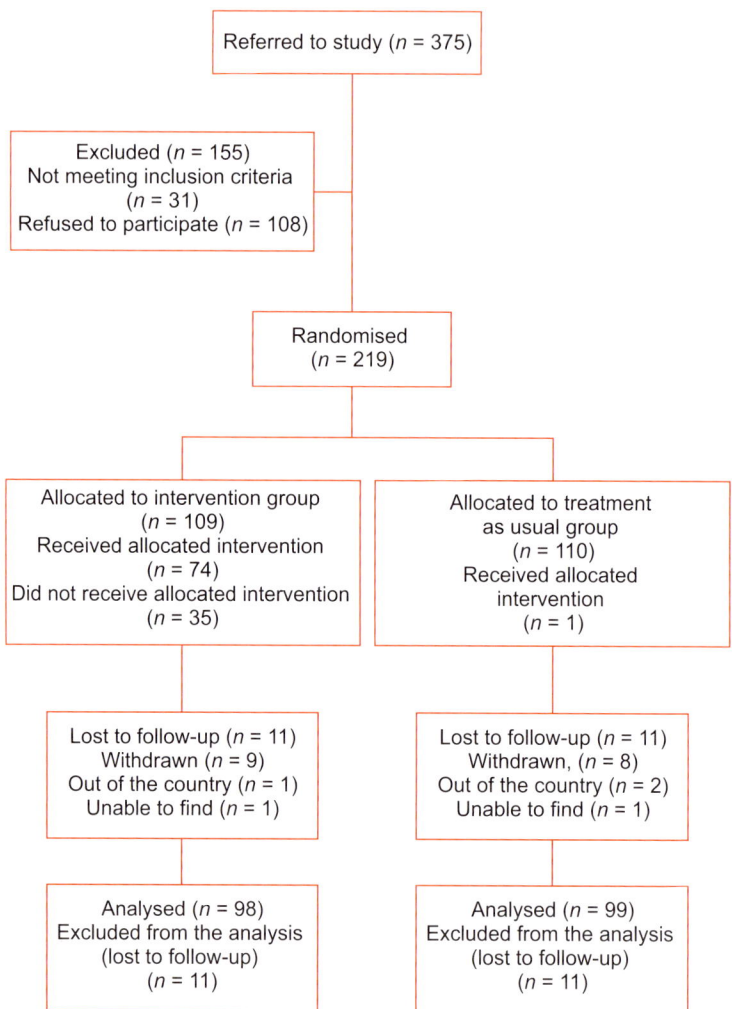

Fig. 34.1 Consort flow chart for SWAN randomised controlled trial of supported employment (Howard et al., 2010).

An example of the project flow information from a randomised controlled trial of supported employment for people with severe mental health conditions is shown in Fig. 34.1, in the CONSORT format.

As you read the paper, pay attention both to what is being said in the paper and how it is being said. From time to time, step back a little and think about how the paper is written. Is this paper an example of good or poor scientific writing and why? What can you learn from this paper about how you may approach writing research papers yourself in future? It is sometimes said that great writers themselves read

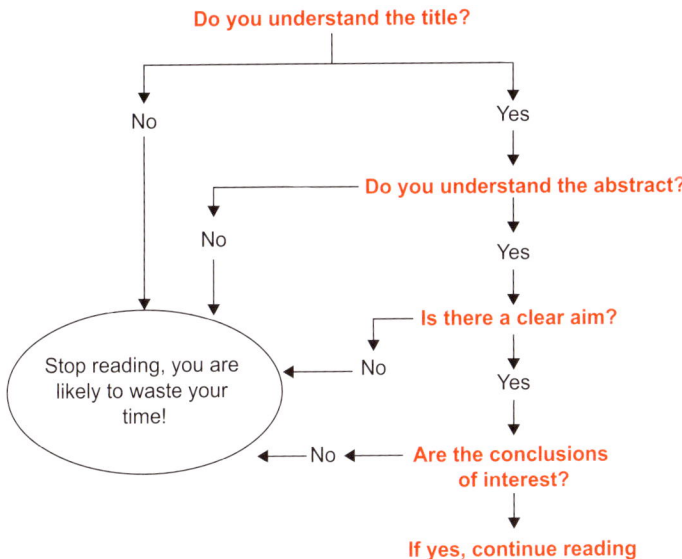

Fig. 34.2   Flow chart for decision making when reading a research paper.

many, very well written, books. Similarly you can learn about how to write research papers well by paying close attention while you read articles that are very well written. Fig. 34.2 summarises the main decisions you will need to make during your search for papers relevant to your interest, moving from the paper to the abstract to the full paper.

Reading the Full Text Paper Section by Section

We suggest that as you read the full text of a research paper you have a type of **internal discussion with yourself** as you go along. Ask yourself a series of key questions, section by section, and try to answer these from the information available to you in the paper, using your judgement on the following issues.

AUTHORS AND CONTRIBUTORS

Who are the authors and where do they work? Is there a clear statement about the contributions of all authors to the paper? Does each author satisfy the criteria for contributorship of the International Committee of Medical Journal Authors? (see https://www.icmje.org/recommendations/browse/roles-and-responsibilities/defining-the-role-of-authors-and-contributors.html). In addition to the authors, are other contributors to the paper named in an acknowledgements section of the paper? Who funded the study, and what other funding was received from the study authors from other sources? Were any 'ghost writers' (paid external writers) used in the production of the paper? Are any actual or potential conflicts of interest declared in the paper? Potentially, who benefits from the results of this study?

BACKGROUND

Given the very limited word count imposed by most journals for the background section, from your knowledge of this field, is this a fair summary? Does the background section grab your interest? Does it sustain your interest or are you bored? Is the aim of the study or the paper stated clearly (usually at the end of the background section)? Is the aim set out in a way (such as in a question) that can lead to a clear answer by the end of the study or paper?

METHOD

Most journals also impose tight word limits on how long the method section can be. Although in theory this section should include enough detail that the study could be exactly replicated later, this is rarely the case, and any replication would need to access the study protocol, protocol paper, intervention manual, or further details of the method by contacting the study authors. The method section should give clear details of *what* was done and *how* it was done, that is, the study or paper procedures used. Read this section as critically as you can. Do the key decisions made by the study authors in the design and conduct of the study make sense to you? Are these decisions well justified? Is the wider study reference population well described? Is the method used to select the study sample reasonable in terms of generating a representative example of the larger sampling frame and therefore can the study results be reasonably generalised to the larger population of interest? If there is a control group, is this identical or similar to the intervention group? Is the sample size sufficient to answer the question being asked? Is there clear information about how the required sample size was calculated?

For an intervention study, is the sample size large enough to detect a difference between the intervention group and the control group if a true difference does exist? Is the intervention clearly described? Is the control intervention or condition clearly described? What scales are used to characterise the participants or to assess outcomes? Do these scales have published and strong psychometric properties? If the scales have been translated, was this a thorough translation process? Have the study procedures taken reasonable precautions to exclude or to identify and assess potential biases? Did the study receive approval from a proper research ethics or institutional review body? Is the approving organisation named, with the approval number for the study? Was appropriate consent gained from all participants? Are there any concerns about exploitation or inappropriate research practices?

RESULTS

For particular types of study, such as intervention studies, was a protocol paper published before the results of the main study were published? For the primary outcomes given in a study protocol paper, are all of these outcomes reported in the main study data paper and if not, is the reason for this clear and reasonable? For results presented in tables, is there little or no repetition of these results in the text? Do the results presented directly correspond to the aims and objectives of the study, and any study hypotheses? After presenting all the detailed results, is the main overarching aim or question of the study clearly answered by the study findings?

DISCUSSION

Is the discussion brief, balanced and fair? Any study will have a number of limitations – are these clearly presented and is their importance fairly assessed in terms of their impact on the strength of the findings? Are the findings well contextualised in relation to previous work in this field and whether these findings support or contradict previous research? Are the statistical, clinical and policy aspects of the significance of the findings discussed? What are the implications of these findings? If we think of a short research paper as being something like a short story, at the end of reading the paper do you feel a sense of completion at the close of reading a well told story?

Recording the Main Points of Relevant Papers

If you want to be able to refer to a paper and its contents in the future, you will need a **method to store the key paper details** in a way that you find useful. Although paper notes or index cards can be used for this purpose, electronic methods have made such data storage and retrieval immeasurably simpler and more efficient. Some early career researchers decide to store paper details in a general program such as Microsoft Word, Excel or Access. Experienced researchers more often use a reference manager program, for example EndNote (http://endnote.com), Mendeley (http://www.mendeley.com), RefWorks (http://refworks.proquest.com), or Zotero (https://www.zotero.org), according to what is available or affordable to them.

Although these programs vary in their details, what they share in common is the ability to search remote databases (such as Embase, PsycINFO, PubMed, SCI, SCII or Web of Science, in the health and human sciences) using key terms. From the list of papers generated that match your search terms, you can then scrutinise their (1) titles, (2) abstracts, or (3) full text. You then decide which of these papers you want to store in your own references database file (sometimes called a library) so that you can access this paper easily in future. Many of the programs allow you to add your own commentary or notes, and also to store a PDF version of the full paper. Before committing to a particular references program, after you have stored the details of a few papers check to see if you can retrieve them easily, for example, by running a search using key words to search, not online but from within your own database file. There is more information on reference manager programs in Chapter 39: How to search for information.

Key Points

- First consider what information you need and if you want to read scientific papers
- Learn how to search for information (see also Chapter 39 on how to search for information)
- Judge each paper in a step-by-step way – to start, is the paper title interesting or important?
- Next read the paper abstract – does this lead you to want to read the main paper?
- In the main paper, critically assess the background, methods, results and discussion sections
- Consider if the authors have any real or potential conflicts of interest in writing this paper
- If the paper is relevant to you, decide how you will make a note of it to be able to easily find this information in future, for example, by using a reference manager program

Reference

Howard, L. M., Heslin, M., Leese, M., McCrone, P., Rice, C., Jarrett, M., et al., (2010). Supported employment: Randomised controlled trial. *Br. J. Psychiatry 196*(5), 404–411.

CHAPTER 35

How to Write a Research Paper

If you are committed to starting or continuing a research career, or if you would like to explore this option, then it is a great advantage for you to be involved in writing research papers. Such publications are one of the most important types of currency in the research world. This chapter offers information for people just starting out in research on how to contribute to papers for publication in peer-reviewed journals. Other related chapters are shown below.

Getting Started

Perhaps the most difficult stage is getting started. While you might want to write a paper yourself, we strongly encourage you to **join a research team**. Most research in the field of medicine or health care is carried out and published by teams of people. This can include scientists with various skills, clinical staff, patients or clients, and managers or policy makers, depending on the type of paper. To start with, simply **offer to become involved** by making some important contribution to the project. This could be by helping to write an ethics application, or performing part of a systematic review by collecting data or analysing results, or by writing or commenting upon successive drafts of a paper before it is submitted to a journal. To a large extent these are **transferrable skills** that you can learn and apply later, even to quite different types of research.

Before contributing to a project, discuss or negotiate if your contribution will be sufficient for you to be **included as an author** to one or more papers about the project. You may want to have this agreement in writing, for example, in the form of an email from the person leading the project.

In some instances you could participate in research and in the production of a paper but there is no way to be assured that you will be one of the coauthors. Be very cautious about a 'We shall see later…' type of answer from the project leader. If the team with whom you would like to participate and be included as a coauthor offers to have you collaborate but does not promise you coauthorship, you might accept this because it will provide you with an opportunity to understand how research is organised and how teams work. However, do not do this more than once or twice because you will have used your time unwisely.

Writing With Others

If you are invited to write a part of the paper, for example, the background or the method section, try to **write together with someone** with more experience of scientific publications, so that you can be coached or mentored in this apprentice role. Do not worry if you are inexperienced. Everyone is inexperienced at the beginning of their career. Do not hesitate. **Just write**. The most important issue is to have a first draft, even if you think this is not very good. The draft will then be edited by others, to bring it up to the standard required for publication. This is one of the advantages of teamwork.

Conditions For Writing and Writing Well

While you write, discover the **conditions that allow you to write** and to write well. Some people need a busy setting, such as a café or a hectic library, to move into work mode. Others prefer few or no distractions and need to find a tranquil place. Set aside a block of time for writing. Some people prefer to do this for about half an hour at a time, followed by short breaks, whereas others need 2, 3 or 4 hours to immerse themselves in the topic. **Stop distractions**. Switch off email, social media, alarms and notifications. Focus on the task. Do not wait for inspiration, **just write text**. Break a large task down to **several small tasks**. If you need to write a longer section, such as the study method, first of all break this down to subsections, each with its own heading or subheading. Write one small task at a time. Give yourself a **modest and healthy reward** each time you complete the draft for each section. Do not expect this to be perfect or anywhere near perfect. Share each small success with your colleagues. Praise your colleagues who complete their writing tasks, small section by small section. Hope that they will also praise you. The paper is likely to contain the Abstract, followed by **four main sections**, usually called Background, Method, Results and Discussion.

Identify the Target Journal

Before you and your colleagues begin to write the paper, **agree which journal** you will send the paper to first. You may be tempted to identify a very high impact journal, even if this is not realistic for this particular paper. But how do you know which journals are realistic? We suggest you seek guidance from the more senior research staff in the writing group for the paper, or from other senior colleagues experienced in publishing papers in your field of research. Look at papers that deal with the same or similar subjects to see how they have been constructed. If in doubt, be a little over ambitious for the **first journal you choose**, but be aware that this will reduce the likelihood of acceptance. There is often a cascade effect whereby papers fall to their level of scientific importance if you submit to journals of successively lower impact factor over time. In our experience, papers generally tend to find their correct level through the peer-review process.

Journal Requirements

Look at the **instructions for authors** for that particular journal. Follow these instructions exactly. If you want to depart from any particular requirements, for example, total word count, **check with the journal editor** first if this is allowable. Note the word limits for each section of the paper and remain within these limits. See if there is a requirement to use particular guidelines for reporting specific types of study design. Many of these are available at https://www.equator-network.org/reporting-guidelines/. Check which referencing style is required by the journal and use that specific style.

Publication Costs

Before deciding which journal to submit the paper to first, be clear about the policy of that journal on **article processing charges** (APCs), and whether you can pay the fees to a specific journal if the paper is accepted for publication. Information about this is available at https://v2.sherpa.ac.uk/romeo/. Check also if your university or organisation has a policy on making publications openly available, for example, through an online university repository.

Who Should Be an Author

Before you start the paper, decide who will be authors. Only people who fulfil the criteria for contributorship should be authors, according to the criteria on contributorship of the International Committee of Medical Journal Authors (see https://www.icmje.org/recommendations/browse/roles-and-responsibilities/defining-the-role-of-authors-and-contributors.html). The first authorship usually brings the most credit and so this is an important decision. We suggest that the **first author** is the person who contributes most to that particular paper, so that there is proportionality for contributions to a paper and the rewards of authorship. In some countries it is customary that the head of the department, the head of the team that generated the paper or the principal investigator of the study is the first author; sometimes the first author is the person who drafted the paper. Whichever of these systems is employed, it is important that you know in advance where you will be on the list of authors for the paper. Many journals also require a **corresponding author** to be identified. This is the person whom the journal will contact about the paper, and also the person who will be named in the paper when it is published as the point of contact for readers who wish to be in communication about the paper. This is often the principal investigator for the study, or the most senior person in the research team.

In some countries, and in some academic specialities, the second most important authorship position is the **last-named author, and in others, the second to last**. Bear this in mind when negotiating the order of names for the authorship. We suggest that all the authors are named in the first draft of the paper, and that the sequence of authors is also set out clearly, using the principle of proportionality, with staff making greater contributions named earlier in the sequence of authors. If it is recognised later that the actual contributions were different, the sequence of authors can be changed accordingly, and it is better if such changes are agreed by all the authors. If many authors make similar total contributions, these middle authors can be listed alphabetically. In addition to the authors, include the names of other people who helped create the paper in various ways in the **acknowledgements section** of the paper – but only if you have their written permission to do so.

Publication Agreement and Publication Plan

For many projects it is helpful at the very start to write a **publication agreement** or contract that sets out clearly how authorship will be decided for each study paper. For large or complex research teams or consortia, it is helpful if the main members of the research team sign the publication agreement before you begin to write papers. After this you can make a study **publication plan**. This plan can be a table that includes a row for each numbered paper, and the following as column headings:

- Paper number (to avoid confusion later, do not change this number)
- Lead person for the writing group
- Other authors or members of the writing group
- Brief title or focus of the paper
- First target journal
- Status of the paper and month for completion of the next step
- Once the paper is published, full reference and DOI identification number

Example of How One International Programme Manages Publications

- At regular project meetings, perhaps every month, the research project team briefly update everyone on progress for each paper, as a form of **mutual accountability**.
- A useful way to **create ideas for papers** is to have time during meetings of project staff to announce such ideas.
- Ideas tend only to be rejected as proposals for papers if they overlap with previously proposed papers, or where the topic chosen is a very low priority for the project.

- Not all ideas lead to completed papers.
- Often, about a third of ideas never materialise.
- Towards the end of the project, proposed papers that are no longer realistic are ruthlessly cut.
- The main outcome papers for the project are given relentless focus.
- This creative process often leads to many good ideas for papers, and to have two-thirds eventually lead to a publication is a very good result.

Structure of the Paper

As you write each section of your paper, remember that for many future readers of this paper English is not their first language. You will therefore communicate more clearly and effectively with them if you deliberately use the following methods. **Use short sentences**. Long and complex sentences can confuse the reader and reduce your ability to convey meaning. **Use short paragraphs**. Many readers will follow the sense of the paper more easily if you break the paper down to small component parts – short paragraphs. **Use headings and subheadings**. Readers can navigate better to the parts of the paper they want to read if you give clear signs of what material is found where, by the use of many clear, short headings and subheadings. Avoid using abbreviations in headings.

Abbreviations

More generally, try to **minimise the use of abbreviations** throughout your paper. If you must use an abbreviation, spell out the full name on its first use, followed by the abbreviation, for example, the World Health Organization (WHO). In using abbreviations in this way you are assuming that the reader will notice the first use of the term and will remember this – neither assumption may be correct. Also, abbreviations can have quite different meanings in different languages.

If English is not your first language, make friends with a colleague who does speak English very well and ask them to **proof read your draft paper for correct use of English**. **Do not plagiarise**. If any of your paper draws from or refers to previously published work, cite that source. If you wish to make an extended quotation from a previous paper or book, you may need **permission from the copyright holder**, and the instructions to authors webpage for your target journal will tell you if you need to seek this permission, or if the journal publisher will do this.

Writing Timetable

When you write a paper, agree a **clear timetable** for the writing group. Allocate different sections of the paper to different colleagues, perhaps two for each main section, and at the start agree a date by when the first full draft of the paper will be completed, and then a date for the completion of the second full draft. Try not to make these deadlines too leisurely nor too rapid. A steady tempo is better to maintain momentum towards completing the paper. As each draft is completed, send the paper to all authors and any other kindly colleagues who may help, especially those with a great deal of experience in publishing papers, **asking for comments**. When you submit the paper it may receive harsh comments from peer reviewers, so ask people commenting on your paper to give you frank feedback. Take these comments seriously and revise each draft of the paper by considering the feedback received and editing the paper. Usually papers improve with each editing round. One paper we wrote for *The Lancet* reporting the stigma facing people with schizophrenia reached 42 drafts before we submitted it to the journal.

Editing the Whole Paper

After the various sections of the paper have been drafted, a single person is needed to **edit the whole paper to bring consistency** of style to all the text. This can be the first author, or a person in the research team who is experienced in writing papers for scientific journals (see the section above about authorship). The first author will usually be the **paper coordinator** who sets the deadlines for each draft of the paper and who reminds section contributors if they are late in writing their sections.

The Paper Title

The title of the paper is so important that we have dedicated Chapter 36 to this issue.

The Abstract Section

For your Abstract, use the **structure specified** by your first target journal. Often this will have the Background, Method, Results, and Discussion subheadings, perhaps with minor variations in terminology, but note that some journals do not use these headings. Many future readers will only ever read the abstract, rather than the full paper. Take time and care to write the abstract very clearly. The aim of the abstract is to encourage or seduce the reader to read your full paper. Be sure that the abstract is a **fair summary** of your paper and does not exaggerate or misrepresent your findings. Ask for comments from within the writing group for the paper for the abstract and also from other friendly colleagues. Write the abstract late in the writing process, after you have written the main paper, so you know what you are summarising.

The Background Section

The aim of the background section is to present to the reader the **most important aspects** of what is known about this particular field of research **before the study took place**. Many journals set a very short word limit (and number of references) for the background section. Be highly selective and only include the most important papers of direct relevance to your paper or study. The background can be organised thematically, for example, about the key topics that are relevant, or it can be organised in another way, for example, chronologically with a time series of discoveries in this particular field of research.

We suggest you see the paper you are writing as a type of **short story**. People love stories. If your paper reads as a story, you will please your readers. Therefore state **the aim of your study** clearly, often at the end of the background section. If possible, state this aim as a **direct question**, preferably one question only. Say why this question is **interesting or important** (or preferably both). Papers that do not state a clear aim or question at the beginning (or that give 5 or 10 questions to be answered) are unlikely to offer a clear answer at the end of the paper.

For the reader who has accessed your full paper, your aim is to capture their attention from the start of the paper, and then to use your writing skills to exert **traction** so that they will want to read all of your paper, pulled through the paper by their curiosity, section by section. Write the background clearly so that your reader will understand what you want to say and actively want to read the methods section next to find out how you carried out your study in trying to answer your main study question.

The Methods Section

To maintain the attention and interest of your reader, try to have strong connections between the sections of the paper, so that the reader has a sense of a clear structure and a strong momentum, flow or line of reasoning of the story. One of the basic principles of biomedical and health care science is **replicability**. This means that a separate team of researchers can reproduce a particular scientific study to investigate if they can achieve the same results. A replicated result gives stronger support to an earlier research finding. In principle, the method section of a paper should be detailed enough that another group of researchers can repeat the study exactly. In practice, journals set such short word count allocations for the methods section that this is very rarely possible.

One way to deal with this is to include, for example, as a **web appendix**, much more detail on the study methods. Another approach is to publish, before the main study results are published, a **protocol paper**. This is a paper that sets out in detail the aims of the study and the methods to be used, and is written before data collection for the study starts. Take care as many journals do not publish protocol papers. An important purpose of protocol papers is to set out in the public domain the main purpose of the study, the main question(s) to be addressed, and hypotheses and the primary outcome measures to be used. Later papers published with the results of the study can then be cross-referenced to the protocol paper to check if all the main outcomes are reported at a later time, and to minimise **publication bias** from reporting some but not all of the outcomes that were set at the start of the study.

The methods section typically gives brief details of **what was done during the study**. This depends upon the study type. For review papers, this section will specify how papers were included or excluded in the study, often using the PRISMA reporting guidelines. For clinical intervention studies there will be sections on the inclusion and exclusion criteria for participants; recruitment and consenting procedures; assessment methods used and when they were used; and the statistical methods used for the data analyses. To learn which sections are needed, look at the online version of the journal you will first submit to, find papers reporting the same study design as your study, and find all the headings and subheadings used in the methods section for similar published papers. Using these headings is a good way to start setting the structure for this section.

The Results Section

In the results section, you briefly present the main findings of the study. Results can be presented in paragraphs of textual information or in tables or figures. Do not repeat the detailed findings in both text and tables. Check the webpage of your target journal with the instructions for authors for the required format for tables and figures. Commonly these are presented in the submitted manuscript at the end of the discussion or conclusions section, with each table or figure shown on a separate page. A table or a figure should be understandable in itself, including all the information shown in the title, legends and footnotes. Note in the text where each table or figure should appear in the published paper, for example, by adding '(Table 3 about here)' between paragraphs at the appropriate point in the results section. Try to base the structure of the results on the aims, objectives or hypothesis of the study, in the same sequence. Start with the most important findings. Report the results of the study in relation to all the study aims and objectives. If you undertake data analyses that you did not originally plan *('a posteriori')*, make this clear and differentiate these from the originally planned analyses *('a priori')*. Many journals have a limit for the number of tables and figures that they allow – respect these limits.

The Discussion Section

While the background section of the paper includes information about what is known in this particular field of research *before* your study is carried out, the discussion section is different. The discussion is where you present to the reader your **interpretation of the findings** – what do your findings mean? This section will often start with a very short summary of the main study findings. Then you can go on to discuss these findings by commenting on whether these are consistent with previous studies or not. In the middle of the discussion section is usually a paragraph or two on the **limitations of the study**. All research studies have limitations, so be open about any difficulties in the design or conduct and how this might have reduced the strength of your findings. The last section of the discussion section often refers to the **implications of the findings**. Depending upon the nature of your paper, these may be implications for future research, for clinical practice, for policy or for teaching. Try not to say simply that further research is required. This is boring and seems to be self-seeking to keep researchers in paid employment. If your results do suggest that further research is needed to take this line in inquiry further, be very specific about what questions need to be further investigated. Try to end the discussion, and therefore the paper as a whole, on a positive note to lift the mood and spirits of the reader who has eventually reached this end point of the paper.

Acknowledgements

Many journals allow a section late in the paper for acknowledgements. Here you can name, if you have their **written permission**, **people who helped you** with the paper. Try to be generous and inclusive in showing gratitude in this way. This section can also include details of the funding source for the research and other funding sources giving grants or resources to all of the authors. Note that these funding bodies can only link their research grant investments to particular papers, as research outputs, if they are named in this acknowledgements section, so try to be inclusive here.

Conflicts of Interest

Most journals have detailed requirements for all authors to declare actual or potential conflicts of interest. Follow these guidelines carefully, and if in doubt, overdeclare any such conflicts.

References

Follow the **style guidelines** of the particular journal you are about to submit to for their requirements of the format of the textual citations of papers, and the style used in the final references section. Check all the references for accuracy. Misspellings or missing information in the references section gives a poor impression to reviewers, and does not convey to them the sense that the authors have given the attention to detail required of high-quality scientific work.

Submitting the Paper

When the more experienced members of the research team agree that, from editing several drafts, the paper has reached a publishable level of quality, it is ready for submission. This is usually now done though the website of the journal. This process can be very time consuming, for example, the details of all the authors need to be entered into the system. Be sure to complete all sections properly.

The Letter of Motivation (Covering Letter)

Many journals allow you to submit a covering letter to the editor alongside the paper. Take this opportunity. At this stage, the only question is whether the editor, or deputy editor, will decide to reject the paper or to send it for peer review. Many good journals review only 10% or fewer of the papers they receive. A **strong**

covering letter can improve the chance that your paper will be sent for review. Make this letter short. Address the letter in person to the name of the editor. Say what your paper contributes to science and knowledge in your field. Explain briefly why this **research is new or important**. Do you confirm or contradict previous findings? What is the wider public health or societal importance of your work? Can you say that this is a very well-designed and conducted study that produces **strong findings**? Will the paper be controversial? How will your paper directly contribute to the mission of the journal and enhance its reputation? If you draft this covering letter, ask for comments from your research group on how to improve it before you submit the letter. The letter is the primary way to initially **sell your paper to the journal**.

Steps in the Submission Process

If the journal rejects the paper without reviewing it, discuss with your research team members at that time (or in advance) which will be the second journal to approach. Often this will be a journal with a slightly lower **impact factor** than the first journal selected. Usually the first author will then need to **reformat the paper**, exactly in line with the instructions for authors of the new journal. This can include a different style for the references, which is often simple to do using a bibliometric database program such as Mendeley or Endnote. Also rewrite the covering letter.

If the paper is rejected more than once, keep choosing journals with lower impact factors in a descending cascade. Eventually you will submit to a journal that does **peer-review** your paper. The journal will attempt to find at least two people to review your paper. A journal may need to approach 50 people or more before these reviews are completed and this can take many months. Be patient with the journal and its editors and staff – usually they are trying hard to ensure that the review process is completed fairly soon. Many journals will have a section on their website to give you information about how far along the review process is. Try not to ask the journal too often for an update.

Very often the reviews received by the journal disagree. For example, one will recommend acceptance and publication, and the other rejection. The editors then need to decide what to do next. Their options are:

- To accept the paper in its submitted form (very unusual)
- Minor revisions (common)
- Major revisions (quite common)
- Rejection (common)

If your paper is rejected and you find that the comments by the reviewers are superficial, mistaken or suggest that the reviewers have not read your paper properly, you can **appeal to the editor** against their decision to reject. But we suggest you do not appeal too often, unless you have very strong grounds to do so.

Revising your Paper

Commonly the paper will be accepted subject to minor revisions. We suggest that you make a numbered list of the comments of all the reviewers. Then edit the paper according to each and every point, because you will probably need to resubmit a **'track changes'** version to the journal showing your edits, as well as a 'clean' version with all **changes accepted** in the manuscript. In addition, you will need to submit a **letter to the editor**. This letter shows the list of all the comments made by all the reviewers (for example, shown in bold or italics), and after each point you give detailed remarks about what you have changed in the paper and where the changes are. Tend to give more rather than less detail. Show that you take the reviewers' comments seriously and you have made detailed changes according to their comments. Accept critical comments gracefully. Do not be defensive in your response. If in doubt, edit the paper as you are guided to. Only decide not to make a change related to a reviewer's comment if you can strongly justify to the editor why you decline a particular editing recommendation. These letters to editors are commonly 5–10 pages long. Although a journal may take many months to review your paper, they often suggest a deadline of just 2 weeks or so to revise your paper. If you cannot revise the paper thoroughly in this short period, contact the editor to ask for more time.

Predatory Publishers

Beware of predatory publishers. They are journals that may have no reputation in your field of research, and can contact you with flattering comments about the high quality of your research. They may indeed offer to republish in their journal a paper that you have previously published in another journal, directly infringing copyright agreements. Very often the only purpose of these **pseudojournals** is to encourage you to pay them a publication fee. Indeed, some of these are malicious journals that will not in fact publish your paper, even if you have paid them a fee. If you are not sure which are reputable or predatory journals, discuss this with senior and experienced colleagues, and be careful.

Overall, learn to manifest determination and persistence as you approach different journals with your paper. Fortunately or unfortunately almost all papers can be published in a journal, but less strong papers will probably only be accepted in less strong journals. To succeed in publishing papers, as well as to succeed in a scientific research career, you will need to persist and persist and persist.

Key Points

- Create or join a writing team to write a paper
- Decide who will draft which section
- Make and keep to a clear timetable
- Decide at the start which journal you will submit the paper to initially
- Follow the 'instructions to authors' for this journal, e.g., for word count limits for the paper sections and style to be used for citations and references

- Draft, redraft and redraft the paper, taking into account authors' comments
- Identify the conditions under which you can find blocks of time to write well
- Most people write best when they stop interruptions so they can concentrate on writing
- Consider from the start article processing charges (APCs) for different journals and agree who will pay these costs if your paper is accepted by a particular journal
- Spend time crafting an intriguing title and writing an engaging cover letter to the journal editor
- If you are invited by a journal to revise and resubmit your paper, take every point made by the reviewers seriously, and give a clear statement to the editor of how you have revised the paper to take into account each comment received
- If a paper is declined by a journal, tend to revise and improve the paper before submitting to another journal
- Keep persisting in revising the paper and submitting to other journals if necessary
- Most papers will be publishable if they are at least reasonably good and, in overall terms, papers find journals suitable to their field of study and quality

CHAPTER 36

How to Select a Title For a Research Paper

Choosing a title for a research paper is one of the most important decisions in the whole process of writing the publication. In Chapter 34 we explain that many readers will only ever read the title of your paper, after which they will decide not to go to the abstract. How can you create titles that hook the reader so that they want to read more of your paper? Related chapters are shown below.

RELATED CHAPTERS

Chapter 34. How to read a research paper
Chapter 35. How to write a research paper

The Purpose of a Title

What is the purpose for a title in a scientific paper? It is primarily **to help you to find this paper** if you may be interested in its content. If you are generally interested in a specific field of research or starting to conduct a systematic review on a particular topic, you need to search for and find the most relevant scientific publications. Such searches are now almost always carried out online, for example, using the PubMed search engine (https://pubmed.ncbi.nlm.nih.gov/). PubMed mainly accesses the MEDLINE database of references and abstracts on life sciences and biomedical topics. The United States National Library of Medicine at the National Institutes of Health maintains this database. To search for papers on a particular topic, you enter into PubMed 'search terms', for example, words from the paper title, author names or year of publication. The database is searched for papers that match your search terms, usually either for words in the paper titles or words given in the 'key words' of research papers.

Therefore when you write a paper title, you **need to imagine the future and to anticipate what words other researchers may enter** into PubMed, if you want them to find your paper. These specific words must then appear either in your paper title or in the key words of your paper (key words are up to about 10 words not included in the paper title but placed near the paper abstract that are likely to be used to search for your paper). The first purpose of a paper title is therefore to allow others **to find your paper** after it is published.

The second purpose of the title is **to be clear what material the paper contains**. Look at the titles in Box 36.1 and decide which you think are effective in reporting the content of each paper.

These are successful papers in that they have been accepted for publication in a strong journal, with an impact factor of 17.7 in 2022, according to Journal Citation Reports, Clarivate Analytics, 2023. Which titles do you consider to be more or less effective? Is 'The Power of Potentials' sufficiently detailed to give you a clear idea of the content of the paper? Do you understand what 'Prefrontal Cortical GABA Neuron Alterations' means? (gamma-aminobutyric acid, GABA, is a chemical made in the brain). Do you know what Sutton's Law is? Do you want to know? A title should tell the reader what the paper is about, and do so very quickly. Many readers will spend a second or less looking at the title in a search engine. Therefore the title needs to be long enough to be **descriptively accurate** about the topic of the paper.

The third purpose of a title is to magnetically seduce or **attract the reader** to take the next step, which is to read the paper abstract. This means that the title needs to induce curiosity in the reader to want to stay with your work at least a few seconds longer. A paper title phrased as a question may stimulate such intrigue, although many journals do not allow questions as titles. Giving the results of an intervention study as the title may reel in the reader, for example, the potentially fascinating: Zhang, R.S., Gast, K.M., 2023. Knitting: A simple and effective intervention for surgeon wellbeing. *American Journal of Surgery*. Remember that you are in effect competing against millions of other papers for your reader's attention. There must be something in your title that makes the reader think 'Yes, this looks interesting'.

BOX 36.1 ■ Titles of Papers From the American Journal of Psychiatry in July 2023

- Isolating Socioenvironmental Correlates of Race/Ethnicity: A Promising Strategy to Understand and Address Health Disparities. Javier I. Escobar et al.
- Sutton's Law. Joel E. Kleinman & Thomas M. Hyde.
- Cerebrovascular Disease and Neuropsychiatric Disorders: Translating Findings From the MRI Scanner to the Clinic. David C. Steffens et al.
- The Power of Potentials. Steven Siegel et al.
- Recent Advances on Social Determinants of Mental Health: Looking Fast Forward. Margarita Alegrí et al.
- Differences in Social Determinants of Health Underlie Racial/Ethnic Disparities in Psychological Health and Well-Being: Study of 11,143 Older Adults. Dylan J. Jester et al.
- The Nature of Prefrontal Cortical GABA Neuron Alterations in Schizophrenia: Markedly Lower Somatostatin and Parvalbumin Gene Expression Without Missing Neurons. Samuel J. Dienel et al.
- Cerebral Small Vessel Disease Progression and the Risk of Dementia: A 14-Year Follow-Up Study. Mina A. Jacob et al.
- Sensitivity of Schizophrenia Endophenotype Biomarkers to Anticholinergic Medication Burden. Yash B. Joshi et al.

How to Write a Title

Potentially enjoyable ways to generate the title of your paper are to ask each author to independently propose a separate title and then for **members of the paper writing group to debate which has most merits**, or to combine elements from different titles to produce a better one. More often though, writing the title is more prosaic in that the first (lead) author makes an initial draft and asks for comments from the other authors. We prefer titles that have the following characteristics:

- Relatively short
- Full of relevant searchable words
- Include words that are not ambiguous
- Specific for time and place of the study
- Say what study design was used
- Give brief details about the type of study results or outcomes that are reported

Consider the paper abstract in Exercise 36.1 and compose a title for this paper.

This is a paper by Louise Howard and colleagues (2010. British Journal Psychiatry 2010, 196, 404–411) and after a great deal of debate by the authors (including GT) the final paper title chosen was 'Supported employment: randomised controlled trial'. This is short, but do you think that this is too short?

Next look at the abstract shown in Exercise 36.2 and draft a title for this paper.

The title that Flores-Ramos and colleagues decided on was 'Association between depressive symptoms and reproductive variables in a group of perimenopausal

Exercise 36.1　Create a Strong Title For a Paper From This Abstract

BACKGROUND: There is evidence from N. American trials that supported employment using the individual placement and support (IPS) model is effective in helping individuals with severe mental illness gain competitive employment. There have been few trials in other parts of the world.

AIMS: To investigate effectiveness and cost-effectiveness of IPS in the UK.

METHOD: Individuals with severe mental illness in South London, UK were randomised to IPS or local traditional vocational services.

RESULTS: Two hundred and nineteen participants were randomised, and 90% assessed 1 year later. There were no significant differences between the treatment as usual and intervention groups in obtaining competitive employment (13% in the intervention group and 7% in controls; risk ratio 1.35, 95% CI 0.95–1.93, $P = 0.15$).

CONCLUSIONS: There was no evidence that IPS was of significant benefit in achieving competitive employment for people in London at 1-year follow-up, which may reflect suboptimal implementation. Implementation of IPS can be challenging in the UK context where IPS is not structurally integrated with mental health services, and economic disincentives may lead to lower levels of motivation in individuals with severe mental illness and psychiatric professionals.

Exercise 36.2 Create a Strong Title For a Paper From This Abstract

- The aim of this study was to explore the association between depressive symptoms and some variables related to reproductive life, such as history of premenstrual dysphoric disorder (PMDD), antecedent of postpartum depression (PPD), previous use of hormonal contraceptives, and current hot flushes, in a group of perimenopausal women attending a menopause clinic.
- Perimenopausal women, 45 to 55 years old, who had not received hormonal replacement therapy and/or psychotropic medication, were invited to participate in this study. A total of 141 perimenopausal women were included; we obtained their psychiatric and gynaecological data, and we evaluated their depressive symptomatology using the CES-D scale.
- There were a significantly higher number of cases of previous depressive episodes and PMDD and PPD history in depressed patients compared with nondepressed women, and prevalence of current hot flushes was similar between depressed and nondepressed women. Patients with a PMDD history were more likely to have experienced previous depressive episodes, a PPD history and high levels of depression. Variables associated with the level of depression were a previous history of PMDD, current hot flushes, and previous depressive episodes.
- The occurrence of perimenopausal depression is related to a previous history of PMDD, PPD, and depressive episodes; hot flushes only increase the severity of the depressive episode.

women attending a menopause clinic in Mexico City'. Note that this is a much longer title than in the first exercise and includes details of the clinical condition, sample, type of treatment facility, and study country. Do you like to see this level of detail in a paper?

Key Points

Very good titles are very difficult to write. We suggest the following, sometimes contradictory, guidelines in deciding what your paper title will be:
- The title should contain a balance between brevity and descriptive wordiness.
- The title should be factually precise to allow search engines to find your paper.
- The title should entice the reader to read more, that is, the abstract.
- The title should be short and long, boring and fascinating!

Resources

On key words:
    https://scientific-publishing.webshop.elsevier.com/manuscript-preparation/how-choose-keywords-manuscript/

CHAPTER 37

How to Apply For a Post

Your career is likely to consist of a series of posts that you hope will allow you to make progress with your ambitions. In other chapters (see below) we offer information that can help you to be successful in finding new jobs. In this chapter we discuss directly how to apply for a new post or position.

RELATED CHAPTERS

Decide Which Post You Will Apply For and Get the Background Information You Need

Before you spend any time on preparing an application for a particular post, **think carefully about whether this is the right post for you** and if this is the right time. Step back from the detail of the post for a moment and reflect on your life and your career as a whole. Consider the issues we discuss in Chapter 41 on deciding your priorities in life. In your next post do you want to work full-time or part-time? Will you want or need to have a break after your current job before starting the next? What can you afford to do? Is the position you are considering in your current town or city or would you need to move a long distance? What personal or family responsibilities do you have and what would change if you took this new post? What do your partner or friends think about you moving away? Is this the right time for a change? Is your current post time limited? Do you have to change now? Are you still learning in this position? Do you enjoy the work and is it rewarding? Will this job lead to local promotion or career development options?

On the other side of the coin, is the new post you are considering a **close fit to your career aims**? Are you clear about what these aims are? Is this a rare opportunity that only arises occasionally or, indeed, may never again be open to you? Would the new post challenge you to widen or deepen your experience, or give you a greater (and more difficult) level of responsibility? Do you know about the working environment there – is it challenging and/or supportive? Do you know or can you contact people working there now, or who were recently working there, to try to find out confidentially what the setting and the team are actually like? How encouraging or discouraging are the senior staff to junior colleagues? In short, if you are considering a major change to your role or where you work and to your family circumstances, take some time to do your homework and then to decide if, on balance, this is a post you do really want. If this is a difficult decision, tend to pause and discuss with your close family and friends, to guide you in your decision.

Understanding How to Apply For the Post

Once you commit to applying for a particular post, then **give it everything**. Find out which details are available to you about the post and about how to apply. Read this information three times to be sure that you understand every detail of the application process. If anything is unclear, for example, the level of detail needed in a curriculum vitae (CV), or the application deadline, contact the recruitment office or person to clarify these important issues. If interview dates have been set, check you can attend then, or change your plans to make this possible.

Preparing Your Application

If there is an application form, **fill in every relevant section**. Do not leave any section empty. If a section is not relevant or applicable, write this in those sections. Give as much information as you can in each section to strengthen your application. If this is an attractive post there may be many applicants. How do you stand out from most of the others? If you can, add brief supplementary materials such as your full CV. Follow the application instructions precisely.

Prepare all the documents as far **in advance of the deadline** as you can. Ask knowledgeable friends or friendly colleagues to comment on your draft application and help you to identify any ambiguities or weaknesses. If you need to identify referees on the application form, ask them individually if they can offer you a reference for this particular post. Find out if you can visit the organisation advertising the post before you submit your application. If you have genuine questions about the post that are not clear in the notification, try to ask these to a senior person during the visit, or in writing before you apply. Be aware that some organisations will not allow visits or initial contacts. As you prepare your application, think about the post from the point of view of the employer. Think not only about what you will gain from the post, but also what skills and strengths you will bring to your new team. Make several drafts of your application – usually it will improve with each revision. Ask someone you trust to check your drafts for errors.

References, Testimonials and Characteristics

Many job applications will require you to name a number of senior people who are familiar with you and your work who can make a written statement about your suitability for a particular post. These can be called letters of recommendation. If the letter prepared for the new employing organisation is not copied to the applicant, this is called a reference. If it is copied to the applicant it is called a testimonial. We strongly suggest that the **applicant asks each potential referee** if they are able to provide a reference for each particular job application. It will help the referee if the applicant also provides the referee with an up-to-date CV so that their reference can include details of all relevant strengths of the applicant. Check that you provide the current, accurate contact details, such as the email address, of the referee. We suggest that you ask for references either from formal managers or supervisors, or from informal senior staff, such as teachers who have been in touch with you only during the last year or two and who can therefore comment on your recent work and skills.

Preparing Your Job Application

Good practice example: Find out as much about the post as you can, and tailor your application precisely to the key skills, attributes or criteria that the employer wants to see in the successful applicant

Bad practice example: Do not overexaggerate your skills or competence in your application, and don't describe what you want to take from the post, rather than what you can bring or contribute to that organisation

Submitting Your Application

Submit your application before, and preferably well before, the deadline. It sometimes happens that computer systems crash just before a deadline if many people apply for the same position. Anticipate and avoid this as it could stop your application. Ask for a confirmation of receipt so that you know your application has arrived safely. Be aware that many organisations only contact applicants whom they want to interview, and they do not send out a 'not successful on this occasion' letter to people they do not want to see. Unfortunately, you can do nothing about this, but at least be sure that they did receive your application. If the advertisement does not say when interviews will take place, you can wait a week or two after the application deadline and then check, for example, by email or phone, if they will be inviting you to interview.

Understanding the Outcome

If you have passed the initial application stage, look at Chapter 18 on *How to behave in an interview for a post*. If you were not selected for interview, see if you can **find out why not**. Occasionally organisations will give brief feedback, for example, that you had insufficient experience in a particular domain. This **feedback is in itself a positive feature** of a good employer. But much more often no specific feedback will be offered to you from which you can learn. If you do get a letter telling you about the disappointing news of your application, it quite often says that they will allow no further correspondence. Respect this. If they may allow further contact, it is possible for you to contact the recruitment officer and to ask for brief feedback on the reasons that you were not interviewed. They will usually have some information about this in their records, perhaps a scoring system that was applied to all applications. If your request is politely phrased and says that you wish to learn from this process, you may receive helpful information back. Even if you do not, make some time, after a period to recover from your disappointment, to think about why you were not selected. For example, you may conclude that the domains of your clinical and research experience were strong, but that you were weaker in terms of teaching or leadership. If you can identify parts of your own portfolio of skills that need to be strengthened, go on to see how you can remedy this and make practical arrangements to do so. Be active in gradually accumulating more and more transferrable skills that will make your applications for new posts in the future even stronger.

Key Points

- First of all, pause to check that this new post is what you really do want
- Discuss with friends and family the implications for your relationships if you are successful in your application
- Before writing your application, find out as much as you can about the profile of a successful candidate
- Write your application to directly address the required and desired criteria for the post
- Emphasise in your application how you stand out from the majority of applicants
- Stress the skills and strengths you can bring to the new organisation
- Seek comments on your application drafts and take these seriously
- If your application is not successful this time, what can you learn from the process?

Resources

Useful sources of templates for formal documents, such as letters of recommendation include:
- **Microsoft Office Templates:** Offers a wide range of templates for various types of documents, including formal letters. You can find templates for letters of recommendation, business letters, cover letters and more on their official website. Simply visit the Microsoft Office Templates page and search for the type of letter you need.

- **Template.net:** Provides a variety of free templates for different types of documents, including formal letters. You can browse their collection of letter templates, which includes formats for letters of recommendation, business correspondence, job application letters and more. They offer editable templates in various file formats such as Word, PDF, and Google Docs.
- **Canva:** Offers a range of customisable templates for various types of documents, including formal letters. Although primarily known for its graphic design capabilities, Canva also provides templates for letters of recommendation, cover letters, resignation letters and other formal correspondence. You can customise these templates to suit your needs and preferences.

CHAPTER 38

How to Select a Topic For Research

The decision to become engaged in research and the process of selection of the topic or subject of research will vary with the progress of your career, from being at the beginning of your training as a professional, to being a fully trained expert with larger-scale responsibilities such as running a department. This chapter offers guidance on how to choose topics for your research.

RELATED CHAPTERS

Chapter 20. How to present a proposal for funding
Chapter 34. How to read a research paper
Chapter 35. How to write a research paper
Chapter 36. How to select a title for a research paper
Chapter 39. How to search for information

In the early days of one's training, engagement in research should be seen as an **opportunity to learn and build one's career and position**. Time is precious and so the first question one should ask is whether engagement in research may contribute to one's career, for example, by adding a publication to one's curriculum vitae, or by gaining access to a network of colleagues engaged in a research project. It might also be that the senior investigators of a particular project have a lot of influence on the future career options of their collaborators. Joining them, regardless of the type of contribution one could make to a particular research project, may open doors and facilitate promotion. In such an instance it is **irrelevant what role** the young researcher will play: the main gain is **being in the company of decision makers**.

There are also other reasons why one might wish to do research, still without expecting to make a discovery. Thus it might be that participation in a project will make one **learn how to use a particular method** or technological process, or how to apply a particular technique.

It is of course attractive to become engaged in operational research, the results of which can be applied rapidly, making the life of patients more tolerable or rendering the function of the department in which one works more effective and efficient. Research can also serve as a **tool to break boredom**, open new vistas, and help expand one's horizon, while **strengthening the image and profile** of the trainee who not only performs clinical work, but who is already involved in research.

The crucial question that must be answered before engagement in research (or for that matter any activity other than those required in training and by the specification of duties in a department) is the **cost of that engagement on one's time**. If participation in a research project will eat up all the time left after clinical and training obligations have been met, it is wise to postpone engagement in research. Free time is important – not only to prevent burn-out, but also to invest in building one's social network, including an investment of time to plan ahead for both your life and your career.

In thinking about the **time that research might take up**, the first question should be whether duties related to the study will take much '**personal' time** – time that can be used to see friends, read, go to a movie or plant flowers. If too many things that have been the content of personal time have to be sacrificed, it is wise to postpone engagement in research. An important consideration in thinking about this is whether the time that will be consecrated to research is fixed (e.g., every morning at 9:00 a.m.) or not. Having more **flexibility in time** for research makes the management of time easier and the impact on personal time less heavy.

Another consideration is whether the **engagement can be completed** before one will have to change the work position or place (e.g., to spend time on another ward that is part of the training rotation). If this is the case, it is wise to look for a different research project that will not continue after the end of a particular part of your training.

Then there are questions about the '**fringe benefits**' of participation in a research project. An important one for young investigators is whether the study will allow them to **learn a research method** or investigation technique while gathering data for the research project in which they are engaged. Being familiar with a technique of investigation **opens doors to other projects** and can be a major benefit of taking part in the research.

It is also useful to consider whether participation in a research project will **engender expenses**, for example, for travel to where the research is taking place, or to buy some of the necessities for the study.

A particularly important question is whether the **study protocol** includes a portion that **specifies the roles that the researchers will play, how their work will be recognised** and what will happen if there are problems with the management of the study. A protocol defining the roles of the collaborators in the research, their duties and authority is usually produced at the start of the study, and it is important to take cognisance of one's **rights and duties** at the beginning of a research project in which you invest yourself.

There are also questions about the topic of the study. For a young investigator it is useful to be engaged in projects that are 'in the wind', that is, **topics that are popular and fashionable** – interesting for the scientific community and likely to be useful for patient care or in pursuing some other noble goal.

Studies that create a **well-studied group who might be reinvestigated later** can be of particular value further on in one's career. To make certain that this value can be used, it is important to include a clear section in the study protocol of the investigation specifying who will be allowed to have **access to data** and for how long. Another special value of a study is the **involvement of other centres** – within the country and abroad – because it creates opportunities to meet colleagues elsewhere, learn from them, and participate in work that they might be undertaking in the future.

We suggest that you consider using the **Sartorius Study Scale** (see Appendix 38.1) to assess whether it is helpful to you to be engaged in research at this point in time. In this content, undertaking research means being engaged in a research study.

Finally, it is important to reemphasise that the attractiveness of participation in research at the beginning of one's career is different from that at a more senior level. Early in one's career, participation in research should open doors, provide knowledge about using research techniques, and enable learning about how to work with others. The topic or subject of the research is of secondary interest at that point; but it will become central at a later stage of one's development.

APPENDIX 38.1 ■ Sartorius Study Scale to Decide Whether to Do Research

	Options	Score
Section 1. Reasons for the study. Why do research at this point in time?		
1. Contributes to career (e.g., through a publication)	Yes – 1 No – 0	
2. Opens the door to a network of nice people	Yes – 1 No – 0	
3. Opens the door to a powerful team	Yes – 1 No – 0	
4. Answers a question of interest	Yes – 1 No – 0	
5. Helps in learning the use of a technique	Yes – 1 No – 0	
6. Could be beneficial to patients now	Yes – 1 No – 0	
7. Contributes to your image and reputation	Yes – 1 No – 0	
8. Supervisor requires that it is done	Yes – 1 No – 0	
9. Opens the door to new avenues of employment	Yes – 1 No – 0	
10. Breaks boredom	Yes – 1 No – 0	
Section 2. Time required for the study		
11. The research will not take up much personal time	Yes – 1 No – 0	
12. Little will have to be sacrificed to do the research	Yes – 1 No – 0	
13. The research will be completed before I leave and change position	Yes – 1 No – 0	
14. It is possible to decide when to work on this research (e.g., during weekends or evenings)	Yes – 1 No – 0	

(Continued)

APPENDIX 38.1 ■ Sartorius Study Scale to Decide Whether to Do Research—cont'd

	Options	Score

Section 3. Feasibility

15. The research uses methods that can be learned quickly — Yes – 1 / No – 0

16. The research can be completed even if some participants drop out — Yes – 1 / No – 0

17. The research can be incorporated into the normal work routine — Yes – 1 / No – 0

18. There is a clear statement of roles and responsibilities (e.g., who decides on what, who will coauthor the publication) — Yes – 1 / No – 0

19. The research will not engender personal expenses — Yes – 1 / No – 0

20. There is a faint chance that some money will become available for the research — Yes – 1 / No – 0

21. There is an agreement that makes it possible to have access to data for further publications — Yes – 1 / No – 0

22. The research does not present any danger (e.g., of infection) in the investigation — Yes – 1 / No – 0

Section 4. The topic

23. The topic is fashionable — Yes – 1 / No – 0

24. The study could be continued later (e.g., by a follow-up of the persons examined) — Yes – 1 / No – 0

25. The main question that the study aims to answer is clear and can be easily communicated to others — Yes – 1 / No – 0

26. Publication is likely to be easy — Yes – 1 / No – 0

27. The study will involve several (international) sites — Yes – 1 / No – 0

Scoring guide
The maximum score is 27.
A score of less than 10 indicates that it is not useful to do research at this point in time.
Priority should be given to studies with a higher score.

Key Points

- At an early career stage, research is an opportunity to learn and build one's career and position
- At this early stage, the topic of research and the role played are less important than later in one's career
- Research can give you opportunities to learn new skills, research methods and techniques
- Research can also strengthen one's career image and professional profile

- Consider also the likely costs of engaging in research on your work and personal life
- Try to find research projects that give you flexibility on when you can work, and that will be completed before you move on to your next post
- Assess whether the research project will incur costs for you and if you can afford these
- Check if you are clear about your rights and responsibilities within the project
- Try to clarify if you will have access to the study dataset in the future, for example, for a follow-up study
- See whether the study is linked with other research sites that you can visit and learn from

CHAPTER 39

How to Search For Information

Many of us spend a large amount of our time using computers, tablets, phones or other devices. Often, we are searching for answers even if our questions are not entirely clear. Here we focus on how to search for information that will support your clinical, research or other professional duties. Chapters on related issues are shown below. In this chapter we do not address more specialised and technical issues, such as how to carry out a systematic review.

RELATED CHAPTERS

Identify and Refine the Question

One useful way to search for information that you want is to **frame the search as a question**. The search then consists of a process to identify information to answer your question. We suggest that you try to make your search question as specific as possible. If we imagine that you work in a clinical setting, for example, you may need to treat a patient who has been admitted to hospital with severe and suicidal depression. The patient also has severe rheumatoid arthritis (RA), and indeed when she has painful 'flare ups' of RA, her depression is worse. She has been treated with a series of anti-depressant medications with no clear effect. Your question could be 'Which antidepressants are safe to use in patients with RA', that is, which antidepressants have a low risk of musculoskeletal or immunological/inflammatory side effects or interactions?

A simple search using a common internet search engine today reveals thousands of weblinks, most of which are not relevant as they apply to a few of the words in this question but do not address the combination of the two conditions and treatment options. It is more efficient, when using a generic search engine, to be **as specific as possible**. In this case, to include the names of the antidepressant drugs that have been used or you are considering using. This may narrow the field of responses you get. A second problem with using a generic search engine for your search is that it can access millions of websites, many of which include nonverified information, either constituting misinformation (false information that is spread regardless of intent to mislead) or disinformation (deliberately misleading or biased information; manipulated narrative or facts; or propaganda). Without a detailed exploration of the provenance of information that you access, it is very difficult to know which search answers you can treat as trustworthy information. However, the principle remains: **be as specific as you can in the search words or search terms you enter into your search**.

Understanding Peer Review

The principle of close consideration of the work of one doctor by another was described by Ali al-Ruhawi in the 9th century. In relation to research, the beginnings of peer review are attributed to Henry Oldenburg, 400 years ago. In academic work it is now usual that scholarly publications such as scientific journals only seriously consider papers that are submitted for publication after undergoing peer review. This means that several experienced researchers who are independent of the team writing the paper are asked to comment on its scientific merits and judge the strengths and weaknesses of the paper. They comment, for example, on whether the question addressed by the study is interesting and important, the method used for the study is appropriate to answer the initial question, the results are clearly and fully presented, and the conclusions drawn are fair given the results, and on the overall contribution of the paper to knowledge in its given field. Peer reviewers often disagree in their assessments of a paper, so a journal editor will need to obtain two or more reviews before deciding to proceed with publishing a paper. Usually the authors of a submitted research paper will need to revise the paper, based on the comments of the reviewers, before it may be publishable. Peer review is an imperfect way to judge the quality and reliability of the contents of any particular research paper, but at present it is **the least worst method we have**. For most clinical and research purposes, we strongly recommend that you limit yourself to searching the peer-reviewed literature if you have a question related to health care or medical research.

Ways to Access Peer-Reviewed Literature

For people with access to the internet, much of the global peer-reviewed literature is relatively easy to search. One method is to use **Google Scholar**. To do this you type 'Google Scholar' in your search engine, and then click on the Google Scholar link. Typing in the question about RA and antidepressants as we wrote this identified 4940 links, most of which were links to peer-reviewed papers in academic journals. Google Scholar does allow some refinement of the search, for example, 'all papers since 2022', which produced 356 results. For some purposes, for example, if you want to see how a field of research has developed over the last 10 or 20 years, you may leave the year of publication open in your search. But for most practical purposes, restricting your search to, for example, the last 3 or 5 years will give you sufficient material to consider. Owing to the nature of scientific papers, more recent work will cite the most important findings from older studies in the *background* sections of the papers.

The weblinks identified will usually take you to the webpages of the source journals of the papers identified, and this will usually provide you with at least the abstract of the paper, giving you the main findings. After this the situation becomes more complex, depending upon the open access arrangements for each journal. A useful way to find out which journals have a more open access approach is to visit the **Sherpa-Romeo website** at https://v2.sherpa.ac.uk/romeo/. If you are affiliated with an academic institution such as a university, you will have much greater access to full papers in journals than you would as an independent researcher or clinician. If possible, try to establish a link with a local college or university to see if they can provide you with an academic status so you can use their online library and journal search facilities.

Reference Manager Programs

If you want to store information that you find when you search, for use in the future, for example, in writing a paper or a project proposal yourself, we suggest you consider using a **special program called a reference manager**. There are many options but basically these are either free (such as Mendeley) or paid products (such as EndNote, which may be available to university staff without an individual fee). These programs can do several things: search online databases for papers in response to a particular query; store papers that you want to keep for future reference; lead to websites where the full versions of papers can be read; and, for some papers, allow access to and storage of downloadable versions, for example, in pdf format.

Example of a Search For References

Let us consider a worked example to see how to perform these steps, in this case using a program called EndNote, owned by a company called Clarivate. In this example, the aim is to find a recent paper about treatment for depression concurrent with rheumatoid arthritis and insert this reference into a paper you are writing on this topic.

> **Step 1.** The figure below shows the initial search screen when you open EndNote. It is in 'online search mode', indicated by the highlight to the small picture of the world at the top left.

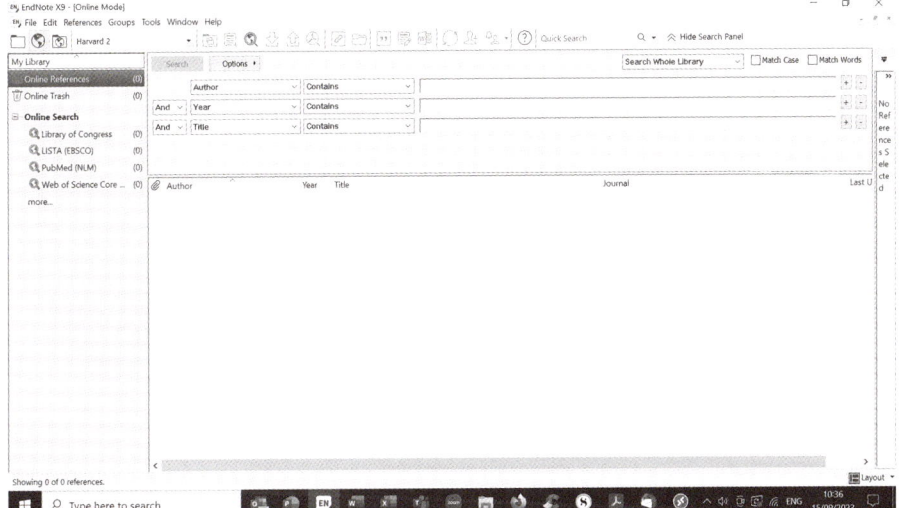

Step 2. You now enter 'search terms'. Choose from the top central fields and select, for example, author, year, title or abstract. You can combine two, three or more search terms, and you can indicate if you are searching for 'term 1' <u>and</u> 'term 1' or for 'term 1' <u>or</u> 'term 2'. In the 'online search' list on the left, choose the database you want to search. Most often we use the 'PubMed' database. Then click 'Search'.

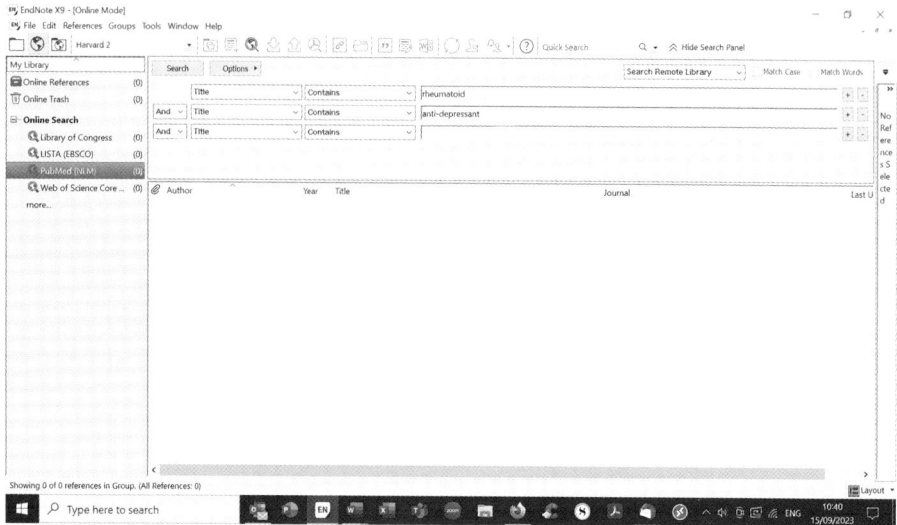

Step 3. In the central area, the program will display the papers that it has found that meet your search criteria, as shown below.

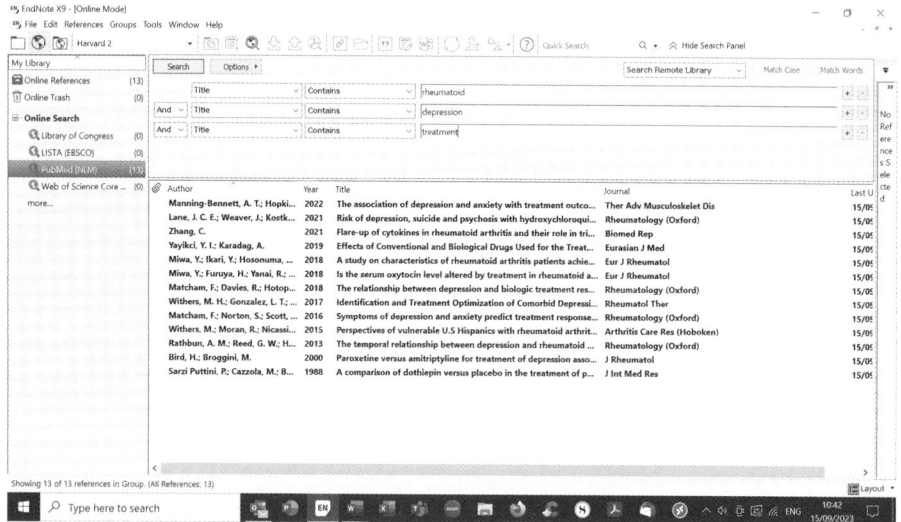

Step 4. You now need to select, from the list shown, the references that you want to save to your own database file of references (which is called a 'library' in

EndNote). You do this by highlighting one or more references in the central box and then, using the right mouse button, selecting 'copy references to' and idenitifying the name of your library to which you want to save these new references.

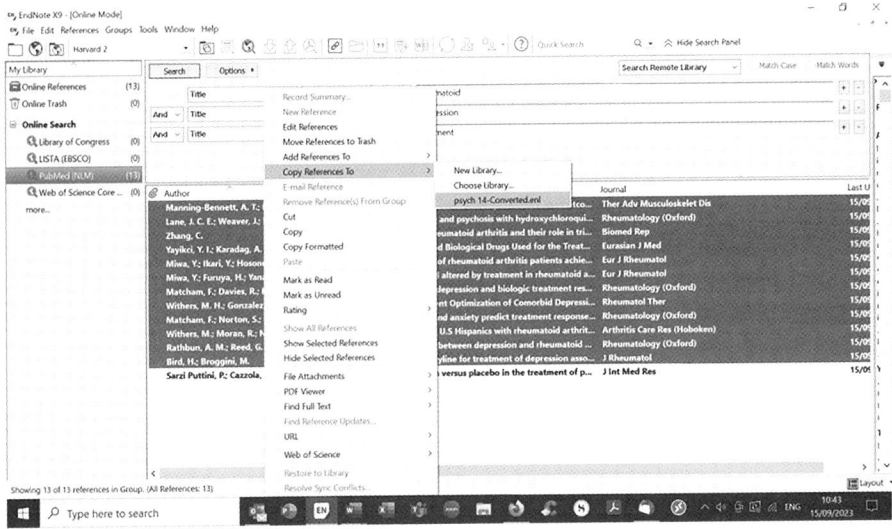

Step 5. To use your library to include references to cite in a paper you are writing, you first need to change from 'online search mode' to 'local library mode' by clicking on the small file icon at the top left.

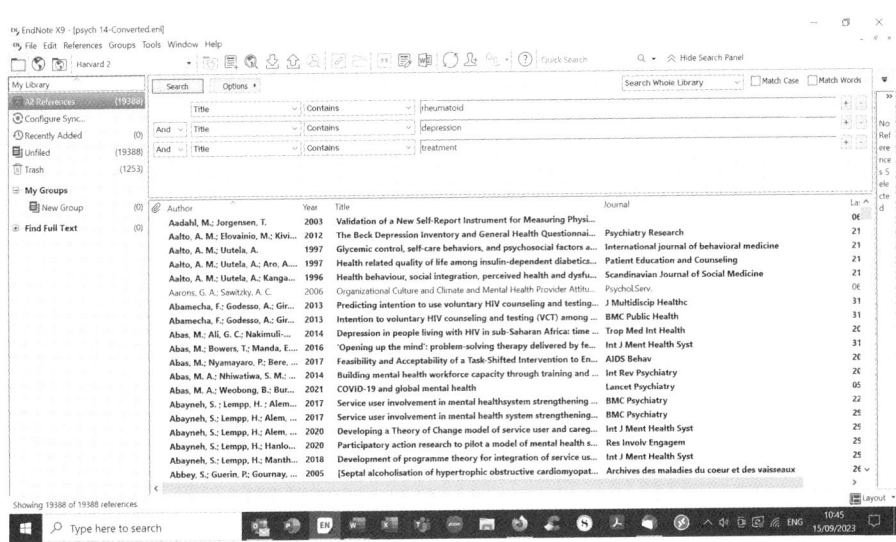

Step 6. Now change to your word processing program, such as Microsoft Word. You need to add a toolbar in Word for the EndNote program, and you will find instructions on the internet about how to do this. You can start to write your

paper up to the point where you want to cite a reference source in the main text, as shown below. In Word you then click on 'EndNote' on the top menu.

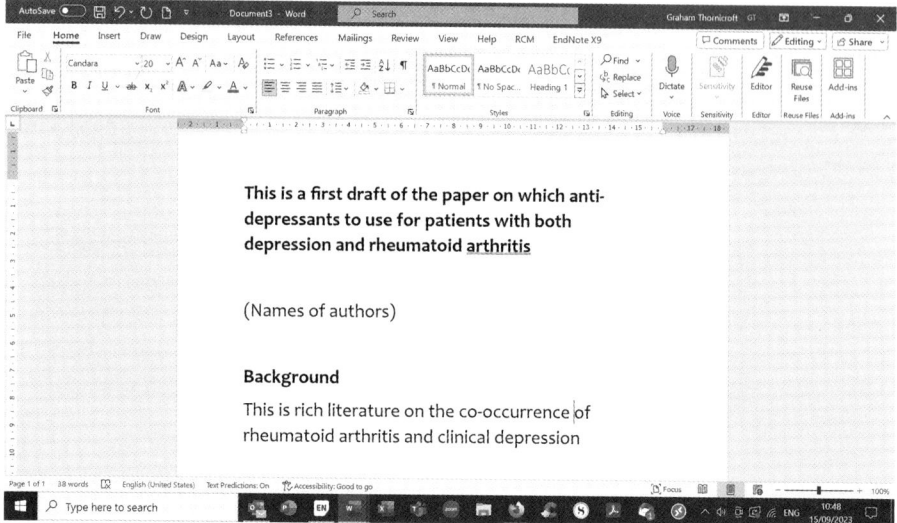

Step 7. You then click the 'insert citation' button, and in the empty box that appears in the new window you type in a key word, such as a paper title word or an author name, and click 'Find'. A list of papers in your save library that include this search term will appear. You highlight the reference you want to cite and click 'Insert'.

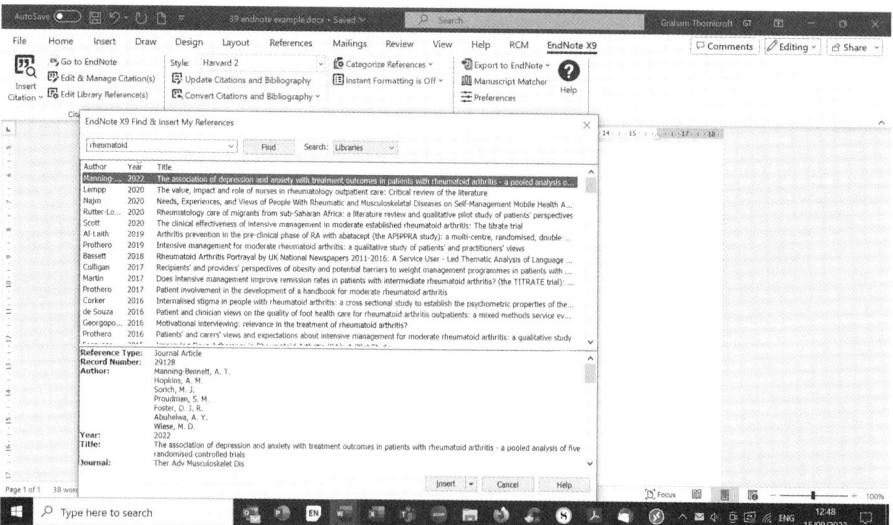

Step 8. You have now inserted a citation in the text and displayed the citation in the references list at the end of the paper. The final issue to consider is the style of the display of the references. In the example below, this style is 'Vancouver',

but you can change this easily by clicking on the menu next to 'Vancouver' to select a different style, and then clicking 'Update citations and bibliography to change the display in the main text and in the reference list. Check with the online 'Instructions for Authors' of the particular journal to which you will submit the paper, for the required reference style.

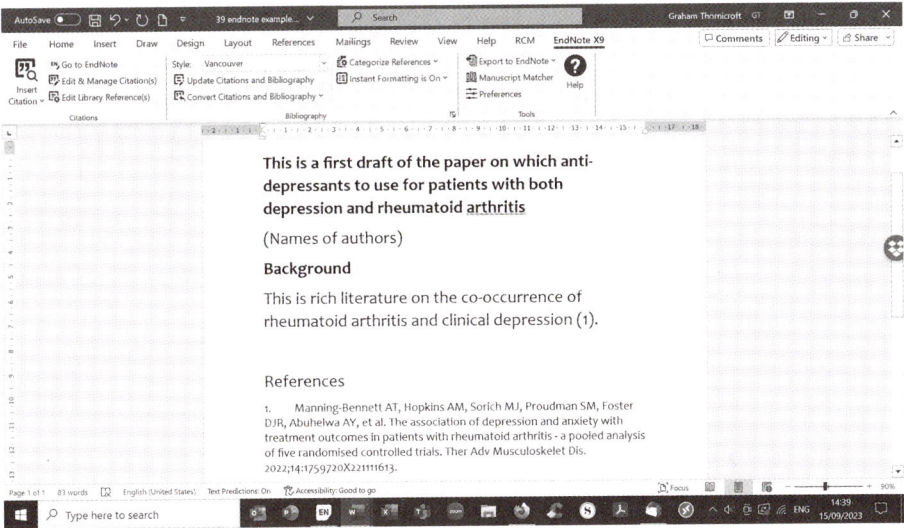

Using Artificial Intelligence (AI) Programs to Search For Information

Just before this chaper was written, powerful new AI programs, such as ChatGPT, Bard and GPT-4, became widely publically available. It is likely that these will radically transform how information can be searched for by people using such programs. Because this field is changing so quickly and it can take 1–2 years from the time a book is written until it is published, we have not included here information on AI programs, which would almost certainly be out of date by the time you read this.

Key Points

- Frame your search or query as a question if possible, phrased as precisely as possible
- For clinical or scientific information that is more reliable, we recommend you search for information from peer-reviewed sources rather than from the open internet
- Although peer review is imperfect in many ways, it is the least worst way we have at present to establish relatively reliable information
- A general search using, for example, Google Scholar, can give you a good initial scope of the material available to help answer your questions
- To be able to store and retrieve specfic references in future, for example, to write a scientific paper or a project proposal, we suggest you use a reference manager program such as Mendeley or EndNote

CHAPTER 40

How to Manage Your Time

Managing time is a skill that can take different forms depending on the person's personality, age, profession and gender. **Some rules**, however, are useful in all instances. Related chapters are shown below.

RELATED CHAPTERS

Chapter 22. How to negotiate
Chapter 23. How to say No
Chapter 41. How to decide on priorities in work and in life

The first of these is to **examine the obligations** that one has and consider each one of them. Any that are ongoing but no longer **seem important or interesting** should be eliminated. Thus a membership of a society that holds regular meetings should be maintained for a subject of great interest. Others whose meetings are attended occasionally, or that do not have any activities that are of personal or professional interest, should be stopped. Regular meetings on a subject of lesser importance reduce the possibility of **structuring time in an effective way**.

Once the list of **activities that are important** for one's existence (such as those related to one's employment and family) is established, it is useful to reexamine it, **together with a close friend or family member**. The **activities that are candidates for deletion** need particularly close attention – often among those most boring there are some that serve to build one's family, career and quality of life.

One of the enemies of effective work are **interruptions**. Some of them cannot be avoided, others can. A good example are **telephone calls**: even if one eventually decides to not respond to a call, the interruption caused by the call breaks the trend of thought and action. It will therefore be better to **put the phone away**, sufficiently far not to be heard during any **activity requiring concentration**. If there are calls that one does not want to miss, for example, those from one's family or children, it is a wise investment to buy a **second, cheap phone**, the phone number of which will be known only to family members.

The second enemy of effective use of time is working with **tools that are complicated or difficult to use**. Relying on computers is a wonderful way to save time if the person knows how to handle them. If this is not the case, it would be useful to **take a course** on using computers and consult others who are good at using them. The usefulness of tools supposed to save time depends on how well we can use them, not on the potential of the tool.

A third area, in addition to tools that one can use efficiently and the protection of one's time from intrusions, is the **clarification of one's priorities**. Earlier we discussed eliminating activities that are not important: what is left to do is to examine which of the activities seen as important **should be dealt with first**. There are often situations in which time is wasted by hesitation on what to take on first, or take on at all. The examination of one's priorities should be a **continuing, ongoing effort** because **priorities change** and **so does the person** who is engaged to deal with them.

The examination of the **order of priorities** and their relative importance should be a daily activity because the situations change, people change and so do the tasks to be done and their order, over time and **in harmony with one's age**. It is useful to **reserve some time each day** to such an examination of the areas of action concerning our existence.

There are certain approaches that are recommended to **save time in office work**. Thus in dealing with one's correspondence it is recommended **never to take the same letter twice in one's hand (or deal with the same email twice):** once the letter is read, the reader should **decide on action to follow, not postpone** the decision about action. When initiating a **discussion, it is useful to define its purpose** in advance, otherwise the discussion may derail and lead to discussion of topics that will take time without achieving much. When introducing a task to a team, it is important to decide whether all those concerned should be present at the same time or be addressed one by one before convening a joint meeting (which can then be short).

Defining the limits and goals of discussions makes them shorter and more productive; this makes it is useful to **spend time defining the goal** and manner of a discussion before initiating it.

When working in a team, it is also important to study the way in which people argue and the topics they are likely to bring into the discussion. **Listing those topics as being important** in advance and reserving time for their discussion may save time and effort.

It is important to organise your diary and time so that you give at least as much priority to spending time on work that you initiate or which is important to you as to time spent with or for other people. Depending on how and when you work best, this can include:

- Usually keeping the first or last **hour or two of the day free** of appointments so that you have uninterrupted time to make progress on your own ideas or projects.
- Keeping one day a week, or perhaps one day every 2 weeks, **free of meetings** so that you have enough time to concentrate on more complex tasks or projects.
- Booking these times into your diary and making these '**appointments with yourself**' a high priority, which are not sacrificed except for occasional and very important alternatives.
- Using these blocks of time for you to be **proactive** in your own work and not **reactive** to the demands of others, and to make time to enjoy being creative to produce your highest quality of work.
- Using some of this personal time to reflect on your priorities and course of life.

None of techniques for saving time can be effective unless you understand that **saving time is not the goal**: the goal is to use time in a manner that will promote **development of initiatives seen as important**. It follows that time cannot be managed in a vacuum: it must be apportioned to action that will **advance progress in priority areas**. Managing time will not and should not result in creating many hours or days in which nothing needs to be done, unless one's ultimate goal is to do nothing, just letting life take its course.

Key Points

- Examine whether your obligations are both important and interesting
- Rank your commitments in order of importance and decide which to drop
- Decide if you can manage some of your time to reduce or stop interruptions
- Only use time-saving tools if they actually do save you time
- Try to start each meeting or work-related encounter by making clear its purpose, and this may mean spending some time at the start of a meeting to define its goal
- Set blocks of time in your diary for work you need to do alone – make these 'appointments with yourself' at least as important as meetings with others
- On an ongoing basis, consider and reconsider your priorities in life

CHAPTER 41

How to Decide on Priorities in Work and in Life

The time of one's life is limited and it is therefore necessary to decide which activities will receive priority. Setting priorities by necessity means that tasks identified as low- or lower-rank priorities need to be dropped. It is impossible in life to actually do all the things you might wish to do – **hard choices are inevitable**. In this chapter, we discuss the basis on which you can make such choices, and how to identify and act upon what is most important for you, both **in your working life and in your personal life**. Related chapters are shown below.

RELATED CHAPTERS

Chapter 22. How to negotiate
Chapter 23. How to say No
Chapter 40. How to manage your time

For most people, the distribution of their time follows the illustration shown in schematic terms in Table 41.1, according to our experience and reports from colleagues in a range of walks of life. We have found that often it is the case that when faced with a series of tasks, individuals do not distinguish between **what is urgent or not, and what is important or not**. Often people respond to tasks simply in the sequence in which they occurred.

Most of the things that come our way are not particularly important, and only a small number of tasks that we should do are truly urgent. Both 'important' and 'urgent' are thus adjectives used to describe activities that will make a significant – positive or negative – difference. **'Urgent' is used here** to describe tasks or activities which unless done without delay will bring harm to one's family, friends, career and being part of society. **'Important' refers** to tasks or activities that make a difference in relation to our lives, lives of our families and communities.

The descriptions 'urgent' and 'important' help in postponing, deleting or delegating activities that are not important and carry no urgency. We propose that you decide on **what is most urgent and/or important** *in your judgement*, taking into account, for example, your own, your colleagues or your family's needs, and not what matters most to the people giving you these tasks. Failure to make these distinctions between what is truly urgent and what is truly important can mean that tasks that are of the greatest significance are simply not done, while **time is spent on what is trivial**.

TABLE 41.1 ■ Distribution of Time and Effort by Urgency and Importance

	Urgent	Not Urgent
Important	15%	20%
Not important	25%	40%

TABLE 41.2 ■ Actions Once Urgency and Importance Have Been Considered

	Urgent	Not Urgent
Important	Do now	Do later
Not important	Delegate	Delete

Having made these decisions, which are sometimes difficult, the **next step is to act** on them, as indicated in the four options shown in Table 41.2.

Tasks that are neither important nor urgent should be immediately **deleted**. By contrast, for tasks that are both urgent and important we suggest **immediate action**. For those that are important but not urgent we propose some **delay** before the task is undertaken later. Finally, for urgent and unimportant tasks, we suggest that you simply **delegate** these to another person. For this to be possible, it is important to have already established good working relationships with members of your working or social network, in which delegation can happen in both directions. Where you may not immediately have a person to whom a task can be delegated, we suggest that you consider the options discussed in more detail in Chapter 22: How to negotiate, such as offering to undertake a part of the task, or to undertake it on a negotiated and longer timescale.

Decisions about one's life and its priorities cannot be reached without considering wishes and duties; circumstances in which these should be performed; and one's motivation and capacity. This cannot be done fast, nor does the ranking of priorities necessarily remain the same over time. A way to deal with this is to **examine your priorities regularly** using time specifically reserved for this, for example, during a brief period of, say, 10 to 15 minutes daily during which one might think about one's own abilities, capacity, and current level of energy or fatigue, and take stock of one's personal and family priorities. We suggest that you consider all these issues on a regular and frequent basis because each and every one of these factors, and their relative importance, can change over time. For example, the care priorities for children will change over time and will usually be more immediate and pressing when they are younger.

A further extremely important issue is to consider whether any **aspects of your life are not in harmony with your order of priorities**. For example, you may discover that the speciality in which you are training no longer brings you pleasure, reward and satisfaction. If so, you need to find the courage to act and therefore to change your profession. A serious approach to identifying what is most important to you in your work and in your life should lead, in our view, to the next step, which is to act seriously upon the conclusions you have reached about your priorities, both for your own and your family's health and welfare.

An important consequence of prioritisation is to **create blocks of time for activities that you identify as of high importance**. For example, if you wish not to be interrupted by work-related telephone calls but do allow your immediate family to contact you at any time, you can choose to have two separate phones for work and home purposes, or even to have a 'dual SIM' single handset that includes two different phone accounts and phone numbers.

Similarly, as we see leadership as an assembly of good practices, we suggest that you create clear **rules for when and how colleagues can contact you** when they need support. We suggest that for staff whom you supervise, you arrange a framework of regular supervision meetings, which you do not frequently change, so that junior staff can rely on having predictable access to you for your advice. However, occasionally issues will occur that cannot wait until the next scheduled meeting, in which case make clear to staff how and when they can reliably reach you, and the times at which you do not wish to be disturbed or interrupted.

We suggest that you make a habit of creating 15 minutes each day, for example, at a specific time such as early in the morning, for quiet personal reflection. This allows time for you to think about yourself, your work and your family. For example, you can ask yourself the question 'What would I do tomorrow if I were invited to apply for a prestigious post in another city?' How much importance would you attach to your individual career aspirations and other needs, your family's requirements, and your wider social networks? How do you balance these considerations if they are in conflict? If this new post requires that you move to another city and your family cannot move to that city, would you leave the family or would you forego this advancement to your career? This form of 'rehearsal' puts you in good stead for the day when such an opportunity, and choice, will arise. In our experience, important opportunities rarely come twice and sometimes require a rapid decision, in which case the more scenario-planning you do, for example, during your brief moments of quiet reflection, the better prepared you will be to make wise decisions.

In general terms there are three sets of activities that should be prioritised by people early in their career: the first is to build a **social network**, the second is to **maintain one's health**, and the third is to **think about priorities**. The latter is to enable you to make major decisions when such questions arise, but also, and this is no less important, to enable you to live your life in harmony with your priorities.

Networks can be created or joined and can serve a number of purposes. They can be a source of advice for times when you are not sure which course of action to take. Networks can also support you in times of need, for example, after a bereavement. A network can also act as a source of social and moral orientation, providing positive feedback or even negative judgement about your behaviour. A network can also serve as a resource to recruit friends or colleagues who have specific and valuable knowledge or skills for tasks that you need to accomplish, or for a project that you need to start. The network can also provide you with protection against harm or against threats that may confront you in life.

In overall terms, it is important to mention that a very important goal should be to choose and undertake one's work in a manner that will make it agreeable and difficult to distinguish from active leisure. Ask yourself the simple question 'What gives me joy?'. What is it I really most enjoy doing and does my current work or position allow me to do these most rewarding types of activity? If the answer is that your role does not allow you to undertake the types of work that bring you most pleasure and reward, we suggest you try to find the courage needed to take steps considering alternative types of work. This may be very difficult if you have a complex set of personal and family arrangements, for example, related to children's schooling, your partner's place of work, or substantial financial responsibilities. In this case, short-term changes to your type or place of work may not be possible; nevertheless, you can plan for longer-term changes that would allow you to find greater joy in your occupation. Any such change requires certain sacrifices, but the alternative may be to spend your active life hating what you do. You being unhappy has adverse consequences for your family, your colleagues, and your own sense of achievement, and means that you will do your work badly.

We suggest that in your periods of personal reflection you consider how to most usefully spend and use your time and how to wisely increase the time you have for what is most important to you. Think about what brings you most reward and contentment, and how to increase the time you spend on these issues and decrease time spent on useless activities, such as hating other people. This wastes your time, as you ruminate about taking revenge against someone who may have offended you. Such feelings will most of all hurt yourself. Similarly, we caution against regret about things that happened in the past that cannot be changed, thus also wasting your time without purpose.

Key Points

- Explicitly consider possible tasks in terms of their importance and urgency in your estimation
- On the basis of these judgements, act immediately, act later, delegate, or drop specific tasks and responsibilities
- Preserve daily periods of time, for example, 15 minutes, to regularly consider your priorities, personal development and prospects
- Use these periods of reflection to anticipate important life opportunities and take account of the various factors that are important to you and could influence your decision, for example, about whether to apply for a job in another city
- Think of ways to save time, such as removing activities that are not aligned with your priorities, or that achieve no purpose, such as hating or regretting

CHAPTER 42

How to Admit an Error or Apologise

We have stressed in many of these chapters that you are likely to work for much of your time in teams, whether you are training or have qualified in your profession. For teams to work well there needs to be a fair amount of sharing of the joint work, clarity about who does what, praise and reward for successes and achievements, and openness and honesty when things go wrong. This chapter focuses on the last of these issues – when and *how to admit an error or to apologise in the work setting*. Related chapters are shown below.

Why Admit to an Error or Apologise?

No-one likes to admit to an error or apologise. Montagu Norman, the Governor of the Bank of England 100 years ago, infamously said 'Never apologise, never explain', and this is sometimes repeated by leaders with the intention of showing personal and organisational strength. So why might you want to apologise in a work setting? In a nutshell – to try *to maintain or repair trust with your colleagues*. We speak in this chapter about sincere apologies – apologies you genuinely mean. We refer to apologies to peer supervisors and those supervised – in all cases, apologies follow the same basic rules. We refer in this chapter to apologies related to the workplace, but you may find that some of the points raised can also be applied in your personal relationships.

In any work relationship there will be times when your colleagues feel that you have broken (usually unspoken) relationship boundaries, or expressed yourself thoughtlessly or hurtfully. This may be intentional or unintentional, but the harmful impact can be the same. The effect is to *put in doubt the viability of a working relationship*. In the health, social care and academic environments, the quality of the relationships you have with your colleagues can determine your job and promotion opportunities, your inclusion in new projects, your social contacts with colleagues and your personal reputation. There is a great deal at stake.

A *sincere apology* first depends on your recognition that you have *crossed a boundary* in some way. You may get direct feedback from the colleague whom you have upset or, more likely, you may receive this from a third party trying to act as a go-between or mediator. Try to take any adverse comments on your behaviour very seriously – they are likely to be minimised and understated. Amplify the volume of the critical comment for your own estimation of what you have done that has caused distress.

If you intended to speak harshly to a colleague, then this was probably mistaken. If you have unintentionally upset a person, you are likely to have communicated in a way that failed to successfully convey your message. If you have negative feelings yourself when you receive criticism or an adverse comment, do not reply immediately, but *pause to let your feelings subside* and then more calmly reflect on the feedback you have received. Particularly at work, but also in other situations, the apology should be an admission of your mistake. It is not useful to start an apology by saying 'The discussion yesterday was very heated and I might have spoken too loudly'; rather say 'I am sorry to have shouted yesterday during the meeting'.

One positive aspect of making an apology is that it can define or *redefine the boundaries of a relationship*, learned by crossing that boundary or limit of social behaviour. A second positive reason to apologise is that the injured party may blame themselves, and your *apology will clarify that the problem was your fault not theirs*. Third, you can do your best to say that you will not repeat the transgression. Fourth, an apology can *reduce stress at work*, both for yourself and for your colleague.

Most people find **apologising hard to do**. There are people who say that they 'are what they are' and that they do not apologise because they behave and speak in a manner that is theirs, for example, they take a pride in being direct. People realise that they cannot behave otherwise. This kind of statement in most instances harms relationships, which change from a productive alliance to a nonproductive mismatch.

You may feel that it shows you to be weak in a context where competence, confidence and strength are valued. In our view, the reverse is true. **Apologising shows that you do care about the feelings of other people**. It conveys that you are capable of knowing when you have done something wrong, that you *regret that you hurt someone's feelings*, that this matters to you, and that you want to mend the relationship. Apologising creates the possibility of improving communication and *reconnecting with the other person*.

When to Admit to an Error or Apologise

In brief, we encourage you to actively consider issuing an apology to a colleague when you recognise, or when you are told, that something you have done has *caused upset or distress* to another person. Without knowing, you may have caused offence in relation to a moral or cultural rule or boundary. Something you said may have been perceived as disrespectful. You may have rapidly and negatively judged without having the full facts. You have perhaps failed to deliver an undertaking. Indeed, you may have deliberately chosen to offend the person, perhaps because you wanted revenge for an insult you yourself felt. *Timing is important*. If you offer an apology too soon after an event or incident, it can be perceived as too shallow or insincere. If you wait too long, bad feelings can fester and mean that your apology is less likely to be accepted. You may also wish to make a *qualified apology*, for example, where someone is offended by what they see as your behaviour, when in fact you did not take that action but are nevertheless sorry that they feel this way. Or you may apologise for an action (or lack of an action) by another person, and you wish to acknowledge the distress that this caused to a third party.

How to Admit to an Error or Apologise

There are no definite rules on how to apologise and how to mean it. But we suggest you keep the following points in mind. Try to show that you accept *personal responsibility* for what you did that caused upset. Make the *apology, short, direct and personal*, for example by saying 'I am sorry' or 'I apologise'. Be clear what you are specifically apologising for. Do not criticise the behaviour of the other person. Show remorse or regret. Say that you *value the relationship* with the other person, you know it has been harmed, and you want to try to repair it. Ask what you can do to make amends. *Do not make your apology conditional* upon something the other person needs to do. Do not demand a counterapology in reply. Do not let your apology lead to a round of criticism or confrontation. Decide if you want to make the apology in person, in writing or both. Try your best not to make a 'nonapology apology', for example, by saying 'I'm sorry if you may feel hurt by what I did'. In your apology *use active verbs* and the *first person* 'I', not third-person phrasing. If you give an undertaking not to repeat a particular type of behaviour, keep to your word. If you are not able to make a sincere apology, then it may be better to make no apology at all.

Try not to expect or demand that your apology will be accepted – this is out of your control. After making your apology, allow time to see how the other person reacts. Did the person listen to you and allow you to finish what you said? Did they show any appreciation for the fact that you have offered an apology? Did they say anything about accepting your apology, or perhaps that they will need time to reflect? Finally, you may have come across colleagues who feel that junior staff can admit mistakes and offer apologies, but that staff in senior positions cannot afford to weaken their authority in this way. We suggest the opposite – that *staff at all career stages* need to be able to recognise when they have acted injudiciously, take feedback from colleagues, *show humility*, and try to heal damaged working relationships by issuing apologies, for the work of the team to go ahead and succeed. It is a fundamental part of the human story to show that people, including you, are capable of change.

How to Accept an Apology

A very useful guide on how to accept an apology has been published by Griffin and Madden at WikiHow. They suggest the following key points:

First, **assess the apology** that is offered to you. Does the person seem to take responsibility for their actions? Does it seem to be heartfelt and direct? Are there any signs of passive aggression, for example, blaming you for the contested incident? Trust your gut feeling about whether the apology is sincere or not.

Second, decide if you are **ready to accept an apology**. What is the context and timing of the apology? Is it too soon or too late? Is the person a habitual apologiser? If you are not sure, give yourself some time. Say you need a period for reflection.

Third, if you decide to **accept the apology**, thank the person, and say you appreciate the apology and that they have admitted making a mistake. Be specific about how the person has hurt your feelings. Say that you accept the apology. Accept the apology in person if you can.

Fourth, put the apology behind you and **take practical action** to make the relationship normal again. This could mean, for example, resuming regular lunch or coffee meetings with the other person. There may be some awkwardness for a period but try to push ahead and get through this. Plan an activity that you both enjoy.

Finally, you have **forgiven but you have not forgotten**. Be vigilant regarding the person who overapologises or who repeats the same offensive behaviour. Do not expect repeated apologies. Be ready to end the relationship if the apology does not lead to more considerate behaviour by the other person. Also reflect to identify if any of your own behaviour contributed to the breakdown in the relationship and what you can learn.

Key Points

- Apologies are used to try to develop, maintain or repair trust and good working relationships with your colleagues
- Successful apologies can maintain effective team working; poorly executed apologies can damage the ability of the team to deliver its work and harm your reputation and career prospects
- Keep apologies short, direct, specific and unconditional. Accept guilt and do not refer to 'perhaps there was a misunderstanding' statements
- Say that you feel regret for what you did and that you value the relationship
- Show humility and be ready at any stage of your career to make a sincere apology if you do feel that

References

Griffin. T., Madden, H., (2023). How to accept an apology. WikiHow. <https://www.wikihow.com/Accept-an-Apology> Accessed on 19.06.2024.

CHAPTER 43

How to Learn Soft Skills

The idea of 'soft skills' has become increasingly prominent in recent years. This chapter offers a definition of soft skills, describes types of soft skills, and discusses why they are important and how to acquire and develop them. It closes with a section on how to demonstrate soft skills, for example, when applying for a job. The skills considered in this chapter are related to the chapters shown below.

Defining Soft Skills

Soft skills are principally skills in working well with other people, in other words, interpersonal skills. Using these skills, you can more effectively interact with others in a work setting to achieve your own and your team's goals. These skills **promote success** for you and your colleagues. Such skills will be a strong asset to you throughout your career by enabling you to negotiate complex interpersonal relationships and build enduring working relationships. By their nature, soft skills are difficult to define precisely or quantify, but they can be seen as the counterpart to **'hard skills'**, such as computer programming or data analysis. Soft skills are **rarely taught** or learned in training, so to acquire and develop these skills you will need to pay attention to them in other ways, for example, by mirroring good **role models**. It is fair to say that soft skills are **more transferable** from one job to another than hard skills, are of **enduring importance**, and are more difficult to learn than hard skills for some people. In our view, much of what is written about soft skills is simply long and unstructured lists of many different types of skill, without any sense of grouping these into related areas of important capabilities. In this chapter, therefore, we have tried to group soft skills into somewhat coherent categories.

The Importance of Soft Skills

Many employers will assess job candidates not only for their capabilities directly related to the post, but also for a range of soft skills that enhance an applicant's ability to work **very effectively in teams** – the ability to contribute collectively, as well as individually, to the workplace. People who do not integrate well into a new work setting, or are not employed after an initial probationary period, commonly fail because they do not demonstrate the necessary soft skills to succeed interpersonally in that setting. Having well-developed and clearly demonstrated soft skills will therefore put you at a **competitive advantage** in applying for posts and for flourishing in your workplace.

Types of Soft Skills

TEAMWORK AND COLLABORATION

Teamwork describes the ability to work well with colleagues to achieve a joint goal. **Collaboration** refers to the capability of starting and continuing mutually rewarding and effective work relationships. Both require a shared commitment to the tasks that need to be carried out. Teamwork-related soft skills can include, for example, acting with accountability, or the ability to mediate between colleagues with differing views, even to the point of conflict resolution. A series of further attributes characterise people with a strong talent for teamwork and collaboration: reliability, trustworthiness, tact, empathy and patience.

LEADERSHIP

Leadership describes the set of skills required by a person who can successfully motivate (or even inspire) and organise a group of colleagues to be an effective team to achieve specific goals. Strong leaders can identify the work-related goal, communicate the goal clearly to colleagues, break down the whole task into component parts, structure the team to work in a coordinated way to complete the component elements, manage and overcome setbacks, and integrate these components into the completed whole task. In many settings the work is undertaken by teams, and so strong leadership is a **critical attribute for team success**. The soft skills of leadership include strategic thinking, time and project management, very clear communication, coaching and mentoring colleagues, timely decision making, and flexibility in when and how task components are managed. A further important skill of strong leaders is the ability to **delegate tasks** to colleagues: to share tasks fairly within a team and stretch team members with greater expectations than they have previously had, as well as support or protect staff who may have temporary difficulties and need a lighter load for a while.

COMMUNICATION

Perhaps the most important of the soft skills is the ability to **communicate well with colleagues**. This is necessary to build good working relationships with team members, give the right information to people higher and lower in the organisation, and explain what tasks need to be done and how and when. Effective communication is vital to building **positive relationships** and intervening when relationships with others, or between others, break down. Communication includes **active listening**, which involves making time to hear what colleagues say and trying to understand their point of view, their feelings, and what does or does not motivate them to contribute to the work of the team or organisation. Communication is sometime assessed **using feedback** to individual staff members from supervisors, peers or mentors, and such feedback can be formal or informal. Specific communications skills include making presentations at meetings; contributing to in-person and remote/online meetings; verbal and nonverbal skills; written communication to individuals and teams; offering and receiving feedback; negotiating; and managing an underperforming colleague.

TIME MANAGEMENT

This refers to setting overall priorities; breaking down **large tasks into component parts**; allocating time to the overall task; structuring the sequence of components; identifying when any aspect of the work programme is not meeting the required timetable and taking remedial action; making realistic decisions about what can be achieved in each time period; and modulating the time and work expectations on oneself and on colleagues so that the pressure is neither too high nor too low. Strong time management will also allocate this scarce resource, taking into account the **importance, as well as the urgency**, or timeliness, of particular task components. Effective time management is vital to delivering tasks reliably in the workplace to agreed timescales. Where there are interdependencies between components in a larger-scale task, meeting such **interim milestones** is crucial to the overall success of a programme.

ADAPTABILITY AND PROBLEM SOLVING

Adaptability describes the soft skills that characterise a person who is able to modify what they do and what they expect of colleagues according to the changing context of the workplace. If a key person in a team becomes unwell, for example, adaptable colleagues will quickly discuss how to compensate for this absence and how to reallocate tasks and timeframe to continue to meet the overall work objectives. Indeed, in many settings, such as a hospital emergency department, the **work challenges may often be unpredictable** in terms of which types of patients need treatment, such that adaptability needs to be a central element of training and preparedness. Adaptable staff can also recover from work setbacks more easily than rather more inflexible colleagues, and may be able to **read the signs of a work situation changing** earlier and react more quickly when unexpected challenges arise.

   Problem solving describes the skills needed when addressing a **new or unexpected problem** in the workplace. It can mean carefully analysing the new challenge, producing a series of options on how to respond, assessing these options, and deciding on a new course of action. Such an option appraisal is often best done in a group or team setting, and effective leaders will create conditions in which staff members can creatively express views or **brainstorm** how to deal with the new problem to be solved, regardless of their status or seniority.

RELIABILITY AND WORK ETHIC

A skill that is highly valued by work supervisors is the reliability of the staff they manage. This refers to a staff member who is true and genuine in giving a timeframe for a task, and who **usually delivers the task well and on time**. On occasion, unexpected problems will mean **some delay** in a part of the work, and the reliable colleague will be able to identify this at an early stage, communicate this clearly to the manager, give a new timepoint for the task completion, and allow the manager to rearrange the interacting components necessary for the whole task to be done well. Managers also pay a great deal of attention to the work ethos of people they supervise. Does a colleague **demonstrate that they are committed** to the overall work and to their job? Do they work hard all or most of the time? Do they offer to support other individuals or the whole team when the pressure is on? Do they reliably do what they say? Are they punctual? **Can other colleagues depend** upon this person? Is their behaviour usually positive and consistent? Is it pleasant to work with them day by day? Do they keep calm when under pressure? Are they aware of what they can do well and what are the limits of their experience or expertise? Can they ask for assistance early when needed?

CONFLICT MANAGEMENT

From the perspective of both managers and staff working with peers, conflict does arise in the workplace. There may be **genuine and valid differences** in views on how to carry out the work, or there can be **individuals whose difficult behaviour**, temporarily or permanently, causes breakdowns in working relationships. An important set of soft skills, therefore, addresses how well or how badly a member of staff responds to conflict. These skills include several of those mentioned earlier in this chapter such as active listening and negotiation, as well as the willingness and ability to compromise. Effective managers can approach conflicts between staff by **trying to understand all points of view in detail**, both what colleagues say and why they say it, and then trying to establish common ground between the warring parties on which to move towards agreement or consensus. Sometimes it is the case that simply making time to listen in full to a person, and demonstrating **respect and empathy**, are sufficient to substantially reduce tension or conflict.

How to Acquire and Develop Soft Skills

In addition to the types of soft skills discussed above, there are others that can be of great value in the work place, for example, being assertive without offending, negotiating, initiating friendship in new settings, persuading, active listening, and starting and maintaining a conversation.

Soft skills are highly valued but rarely taught in the workplace. The first priority is to appreciate the value of these skills to your team and your career success, and to try to find out which skills you have and which you lack. Ways to do this include **formal and informal feedback** from managers, supervisors and colleagues on your interpersonal strengths and weaknesses. Do not just wait for them to comment on your work, but **actively ask for comments** – this information is very valuable to help you improve your soft skills. Try to pay detailed attention to how colleagues manifest soft skills **as role models**, both positively and negatively, and reflect on what you can learn from them. If a colleague needs to try to resolve a workplace conflict, you may offer to assist and learn from this experience. Try to get involved in different types of work groups and teams to see what difficult situations arise; analyse what happened as a consequence and whether or not it was effective. Find **trusted friends or colleagues and informally discuss** options on dealing, for example, with an incompetent or malevolent manager, and try different approaches to see what works. Some people will do this quite deliberately; for example, they may carry a small notebook in which to write down interpersonal problems at work and creatively think of options for managing these challenges. This can support **self-reflection** on the experience of seeing soft skills deployed badly or well at work.

Demonstrating Soft Skills to Employers

Because soft skills are so important at work, if you are strongly endowed with these skills, it is **important that you demonstrate** this, for example, when applying for a post or seeking promotion. You can manifest these skills, for example, by listening actively to colleagues, being punctual for meetings, asking follow-up questions during discussions, being honest with others, being rather modest in some settings, or speaking clearly and usually briefly in meetings. When applying for a job, it is much better to demonstrate these skills at an interview, rather than by superficially stating on your CV that you are a good 'team player'. If you have had excellent feedback on some of your soft skills in your current or a recent job, state this briefly in your job application; even better is to **include an example** of when you used soft skills effectively. You may wish to include a **short section in your CV** that gives brief details of your most accomplished soft skills, again with some specific illustrations, especially those that clearly contributed to a clearcut success at work. For some jobs it may help you to briefly mention your best soft skills in the **cover letter** (letter of motivation). For an interview, for example, you can **prepare two or three short stories** that clearly illustrate your successful use of soft skills in solving problems at work.

Soft skills are therefore the inverse of hard skills – less quantifiable, but nevertheless clearly recognisable by managers and colleagues when you are strongly able to demonstrate your fluency and confidence with these talents. It is also immediately palpable if you are weak in terms of using soft skills in the workplace. They can make the difference between surviving and flourishing at work.

Key Points

- Soft skills are types of behaviour you can use at work to improve interpersonal relations
- Soft skills enhance your ability to work well in teams of people
- Strength in soft skills can put you at a competitive advantage over your peers
- Important types of soft skills include teamwork and collaboration; leadership and communication; time management; adaptability and problem solving; reliability and work ethic; and conflict management
- Acquiring and developing soft skills can be enhanced by active use of feedback and critical analysis of role models
- It is often important to demonstrate your stronger soft skills to employers, for example, when applying for a job or for promotion

Note: Page numbers followed by *f* indicate figures, *t* indicate tables, and *b* indicate boxes.